At Work in the Field of Birth

To Mary, who
played an
indispensable role
in this project!

xo Maggie.

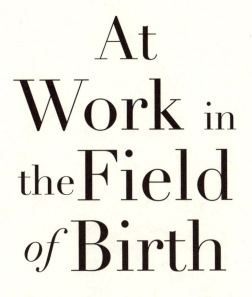

At Work in the Field of Birth

*Midwifery Narratives
of Nature, Tradition, and Home*

Margaret MacDonald

Vanderbilt University Press
Nashville

10 09 08 07   1 2 3 4 5

Printed on acid-free paper made from
50% post-consumer recycled paper.
Manufactured in the United States of America.

Library of Congress Cataloging-in-Publication Data

MacDonald, Margaret
At work in the field of birth : midwifery
narratives of nature, tradition, and home
/ Margaret MacDonald. — 1st ed.
    p. ; cm.
Includes bibliographical references and index.
ISBN 978-0-8265-1576-6 (cloth : alk. paper)
ISBN 978-0-8265-1577-3 (pbk. : alk. paper)
    1. Midwifery—Canada. I. Title.
[DNLM: 1. Midwifery—Canada. 2. Anthropology,
Cultural—Canada. WQ 160 M135A 2007]
RG950.M32 2007
618.2'00971—dc22   2007019253

Contents

Acknowledgments

I AM INDEBTED TO MANY people for their support and engagement—intellectual and otherwise—at various stages throughout the process of researching and writing this book. First and foremost, I would like to thank the women and men who participated in my study. Their generosity of time and spirit made my work truly interesting and enjoyable. My dissertation advisers in the Department of Anthropology at York University—Naomi Adelson, Ken Little and Penny Van Esterik—also deserve special mention as do many other friends and colleagues within and without anthropology including (but not limited to) Ivy Lynn Bourgeault, Robbie Davis-Floyd, Kanmani Guruswami, Leslie Howarth, Pamela Klassen, James Lee, Jacquelyne Luce, Ana Ning, Jennifer Nourse, and Natasha Pravaz. To my family I am also grateful for their support in many everyday ways, but mostly for their love and humor.

The research for this book was financially supported by a Social Sciences and Humanities Research Council of Canada Doctoral Fellowship as well as a number of smaller grants provided by the Department of Anthropology at York University, York University Faculty of Graduate Studies, and the York University Graduate Students Association.

Finally, I would like to thank my editors at Vanderbilt University Press, Michael Ames—whose enthusiasm and steady guidance throughout the project helped make this book what it is—and Dariel Mayer who patiently aided the transformation of this work from manuscript to book in the final stages.

At Work in the Field of Birth

CHAPTER ONE

A Field of Narratives

THIS BOOK IS AN ethnographic study of midwifery in Canada in the wake of its historic transition from the margins as a grassroots social movement to a profession within the public health care system. After more than a century of official absence and decades of lobbying by midwives and their supporters, the province of Ontario enacted legislation that recognized midwifery as a profession in January 1994. Midwifery and childbirth have garnered a great deal of interest in the social sciences in the last decade or so—and for good reason. Midwifery is now being approached from the rich theoretical purview that takes seriously reproduction as a site of cultural production, performance, and consumption. Thus, we may think of midwifery at the turn of the twenty-first century in Canada as a new ethnographic site not only in the sense of its recent reemergence within a particular set of social, historical, and political circumstances that have yet to be fully explored by anthropologists but also in the sense that anthropological theory has changed the way we view reproduction and the body.

In this book I explore contemporary midwifery as a complex cultural system in which bodies, knowledge, practices, and technologies intersect in culturally productive—and sometimes unpredictable—ways. The title of this book has a dual meaning, referring first to the work of midwives and clients in the active cultural shaping of pregnancy and birth. It also refers to my work as an ethnographer in the changing cultural field of birth in Canada. I focus on a number of foundational concepts within midwifery—nature, tradition, and home—that inform the identities and practices of midwives themselves as well as the embodied experiences of women in their care. I pay particular attention to what I call the gender expectations of midwifery, that is, the discursive and performative constructions of gender in the vocation and experience of midwifery and childbirth. In so doing, I describe how the foundational concepts of nature, tradition, and home are being reworked by the practical and ideological challenges of midwifery's new place within the formal health care system. It is a rich and layered story—one that began long before my fieldwork did in 1996 and one that continues to unfold as I write. I begin, fittingly, with a story from the field.

Permitted to Practice

Caroline is a midwife with nearly twenty years experience learning, practicing, and advocating for midwifery, overseas and at home in Canada.[1] Although she is only in her mid-forties, she considers herself one of the grandmothers of contemporary midwifery in Ontario. She was deeply committed to midwifery as a social movement in the late 1970s and was active in the efforts to organize and lobby for its professionalization throughout the 1980s and 1990s. Caroline is now among the first midwives legally registered to practice in Canada in over a century. I arrived in her city by train on a particularly cold day in January and took a taxi to her home. Like many midwives in Ontario, her clinic is at her home on a quiet, tree-lined street. The entire first floor of her house is devoted to clinic space. The reception area is filled with a desk, phone, filing cabinets, and fax machine. There is a small bathroom with "pee sticks" in a jar on the shelf. (At every appointment, women check their own urine for protein and glucose levels.) Down the hall the two clinic rooms look like bedrooms; one overlooks Caroline's garden and has an antique bed draped with a quilt and piled with pillows. There are no metal examining tables or fluorescent lights. The waiting room is lined with bookcases and contains two big comfortable couches. There are posters of smiling mothers and breastfeeding babies, and a bulletin board overflowing with thank-you notes and birth announcements from former clients. A series of striking black and white posters dominates one full wall. They depict portraits of individual midwives from a number of different countries, each with a subtitle that reads: "Permitted to Practice." Caroline herself is pictured in the last poster representing Canadian midwifery.

When I asked about the significance of the portraits, Caroline spoke of the variable and often vulnerable status of midwifery worldwide—from the troubling suppression of traditional midwifery in impoverished countries in the name of development, to the erosion of professional midwives' autonomy in regulated biomedical health systems of the West. At the same time, she spoke nostalgically of midwifery in other times and places, and of midwifery as part of a worldwide phenomenon of women fighting for control of their reproductive health. Eventually, her answer circled back to the place of Canadian midwifery within what she sees as a universal vocation.

> Midwifery in Ontario, and midwifery here in my community
> is part of a larger movement whereby women and their partners
> are brought into this wonderful process—birth—and it's like
> a reawakening. It's sort of a rebirth for them. And I think that
> they start to realize that they need connections and support that
> they haven't needed before. And birth is a great leveler. Women
> start to talk to their mothers. Imagine! Women start to want to
> understand how it has been for other women. They start to think
> that having a baby is not a professional thing; having a baby
> is a connection with other women and other cultures. To me
> it's having a connection with other women in other centuries!
> You suddenly realize that you are part of humanity and that
> connection is a very important one to make. First of all it helps
> you get through your labor because you know that women have
> done this for thousands of years. It also really makes you want
> to go back to your roots and going back to your roots is not
> walking into a hospital to get connected up to a machine, you
> know? . . . And I think it connects us to our mortality too. You

realize that this body—well, you are about to produce this little being that is a part of yourself, an extension of yourself which is going to be here after you're gone and you start to realize that there is much more to life than what you were doing before you got pregnant. Now it's time to become part of creating a better world.

Canadian Midwifery at the Turn of the 21st Century

The portrait of an indigenous Latin American partera next to a Canadian community midwife speaks to Canadian midwifery's self-conscious and critical positioning on a global stage, where it seems that biomedicine reigns supreme and midwives suffer under its disciplinary effects. The images seem to assert a universal midwifery identity and at the same time convey an implicit irony: How can midwives be "permitted to practice" skills that are naturally already theirs? Indeed, midwifery—if defined simply as the act of attending women in childbirth—is a cultural universal.[2] The variation in its meaning and practice, however, is vast. In many societies, all women are still expected to have general competence with managing labor and delivery, while in others it is controlled by a group of specialists, as it is in Europe and North America.

Until 1994 Canada held the dubious distinction of being the only western industrialized country that did not, in fact, permit midwives to practice legally. Laws prohibiting the practice of midwifery first appeared in the late eighteenth century, and by the early twentieth century traditional forms of midwifery had, depending on the region, faded away or been stamped out. Contemporary midwifery is the product of a grassroots social movement that emerged in the 1970s to radically challenge the absence of alternatives to mainstream biomedical perceptions and management of birth. For two decades women in pockets across the country served a small clientele of women and families outside the formal health care system, offering prenatal care and birth attendance at home. In Ontario, they called themselves community midwives. They had much in common ideologically with independent or direct-entry midwifery in the United States and radical nurse midwifery in the United Kingdom; their work was based on the philosophy that giving birth is a profound event in a woman's life, not just a physiological process. Inspired by sweeping social changes of the 1960s and 1970s—especially the intersection of feminism and the women's health movement—the midwifery movement sought to restore the definition of birth as a natural event, to reinvent women as competent birthers and attendants, and to restore the option of giving birth in the home. Their clinical work was characterized by low-tech, woman-centered care.

In the 1980s the midwifery movements in several provinces of the country—for reasons I discuss in Chapter 2—began to focus on the goal of professionalization and the legal allowance of home birth. When Ontario became the first province to enact legislation to recognize, regulate, and publicly fund midwifery as an autonomous health profession, it was a watershed moment in the history of Canadian maternity care. It was hailed by many as a renaissance for the profession and as a victory for women seeking more choices in childbirth. Midwives now number more than three hundred in the province and provide primary maternity care to approximately 8 percent of Ontario women. The Ontario case was the first in a cross-country wave of midwifery legislation.[3]

Caroline suggests that the return of midwifery in Ontario makes sense because birth has a timeless, inherent meaning—an idea that is as compelling as it is potentially problematic. Her posters and her commentary on them speak to this notion of the universality of birth at the level of embodiment. Even midwives less likely to invoke "connections" with women in other cultures and other centuries as Caroline does still remind the women in their care that "women have been doing this all over the world for thousands and thousands of years." "The female body is perfectly designed to carry and give birth to babies," they tell their clients, "so you can do it too." They stress that it is only quite recently that we have taken such a medicalized view of the process and placed it entirely in the hands of physicians in the hospital. Many midwifery clients echo this sentiment. "Home birth is only weird in the industrialized West," said one woman in my study who was getting negative reactions from her friends about her choice of midwifery care and home birth. "Most other cultures would find it odd to go to the hospital. For them, home birth is natural!"

Nature and the universality of childbirth and midwifery have long served as a compelling basis for midwifery as a social movement. It has been successfully employed rhetorically to counter and critique the predominant biomedical or "technocratic" model of the pregnant and birthing body (Davis-Floyd 1994) as inherently problematic and potentially dangerous to the fetus. More than this, the rhetoric of nature serves as a guiding metaphor for women's cultural expectations of pregnancy and birth. How am I supposed to give birth? What will I do in labor? What will be done to me? Natural birth is an idiom for what midwives clinically refer to as normal birth and, as such, carries a kind of cultural weight that goes beyond this term. Assertions regarding the universality and naturalness of pregnancy and childbirth are not just clinical statements but are rhetorical constructions that work to shape women's cultural expectations of birth and of themselves. Thus are pregnancy and childbirth with midwifery opportunities, as Caroline asserts, "to become part of creating a better world"— though midwives may differ in terms of their precise vision of what that better world may look like.

The Reinvention of Midwifery

If the introduction thus far highlights the perceived connections between Canadian midwifery and other times and places in a kind of antimodernist pursuit of nature, tradition, and universality, it also highlights some of the most pressing tensions within contemporary midwifery. In the chapters that follow, I organize my inquiry around key debates embodied in three iconic midwifery symbols: nature, tradition, and home. How is midwifery in Canada at the turn of the twenty-first century still traditional? What constitutes a natural birth from the perspective of midwives and women who have had midwifery care? What should be the role of medical technology in midwifery care? How are midwifery spaces, including clinics, homes, and hospital rooms, produced by midwives and birthing women as ideal locations for giving birth? In critically exploring the discursive and performative uses to which such midwifery symbols are put by midwives and clients, I discover that far from representing fixed understandings of the body, childbirth, and midwifery identity and practice, these apparently nostalgic notions of natural bodies and births are being "reimagined—and relived" (Haraway 1991, 4) by the personal, political, and pragmatic choices of midwives and their clients.

Midwifery in Canada has most often been described in terms of the past—as the resurrection of the ancient tradition of women helping women in childbirth—or in reference to biomedicine—as its opposite. Such descriptions have been symbolically important and politically strategic for practitioners, users, and advocates of midwifery. They have at the same time been identified as the source of midwifery's lack of legitimacy by those who oppose it. In this book I suggest readings of midwifery that go beyond the more familiar content of these symbols and dichotomies. The history I tell is partly conventional, drawing on what is generally known by historians and other chroniclers, but it is also critical, reflecting on the uses of history (and imagined histories) in the contemporary project of building midwifery identity. In short, I argue that midwifery in Canada has not been reclaimed or resurrected from the past so much as it has been reinvented in the present, out of present-day concerns. Despite the unique history of midwifery in Canada and the intensely local struggle for legality and professionalization in Ontario, midwifery today is a product of local social and historical specificity, imaginative connections with ideas of universality, and international midwifery networks and knowledge exchange.

While this contemporary reinvention of midwifery does turn to some degree on its opposition to biomedicine, this relationship too merits a more nuanced analysis. Certainly, the new midwifery's location within the health care system alters its status as a radical alternative in a number of challenging, interesting, and, some would argue, strengthening ways (Van Wagner 2004). Even the notions of hybridity and synthesis, which seek to resolve such dichotomies by presenting midwifery as a blending of science and medicine with nature and feminism, get some reworking in this book. I argue for a more dialectical approach that involves women's agency and pragmatism in a social and cultural field informed by scientific evidence, technology, and modernity as well as the rhetorically powerful guiding metaphors and lived experiences of nature and tradition. Finally, I seek to illuminate the "cultural negotiation of gender" that takes place within midwifery. For embedded within the professional and social identity of midwifery, as well as within the clinical models of the body it purveys, are what I call gender expectations of midwifery—cultural messages about who women are and what they can do.

The Anthropology of Reproduction

It was anthropologist Shelley Romalis who first asserted that "the act of giving birth to a child is never simply a physiological act, but rather a performance defined by and enacted within a cultural context" (1982, 6). Since that time, anthropologists have highlighted reproduction not only in studies of women's lives but also in studies of ethnicity, national identity, and modernity, as a phenomenon in which local and global forces and flows of ideas, knowledge, persons, practices, and technologies come together in culturally productive ways. This literature shows, for example, the transformation of childbirth practices as central to colonial interventions in the name of modernity and civilization (Ram and Jolly 1998; Van Hollen 2003); it describes massive interventions into family planning and maternity care in the name of "development" as laden with Orientalist discourses about "underdeveloped others" (Allen 2003; Van Hollen 2003); it illuminates the proliferating state- and faith-sanctioned use of new reproductive technologies in realizing goals of nation, citizenship, and family in places like Jewish Israel (Kahn 2000); it reconceptualizes pregnancy and motherhood in terms of consumption rather than production only in contemporary North American society (Taylor, Layne, and Wozniak 2004); and it describes reproduction as a strategy in the creation and performance of gender, ethnic, and national identity for Palestinian women living in Israel/Palestine (Kanaaneh 2002:22). In all of these works, the conceptual positioning of women is as agents, as sources of knowledge, actively shaping and reshaping culture and society rather than simply being shaped or produced by it. In this book,

as in these works I have mentioned, it is my intention that "by using reproduction as an entry point to the study of social life, we can
see how cultures are produced (or contested) as people imagine
and enable the creation of the next generation (Ginsburg and Rapp
1995, 1–2).

My analysis is theoretically underpinned by a critical-interpretive
approach in medical anthropology which assumes that "all knowledge relating to the body, health and illness is culturally constructed,
negotiated, and renegotiated in a dynamic process through time and
space" (Lock and Scheper-Hughes 1990, 49). The concept of gender
performativity (Butler 1992, 1993; Stewart 1990) is another important
theoretical tool here, in that pregnancy and birth may be understood
as gendered performances, rather than prediscursive realities. These
theoretical approaches allow me to incorporate and expand upon familiar feminist analyses that identify reproduction as a site of wom-
en's oppression and, therefore, a potential site of women's emancipation or empowerment. My central theoretical argument in this book
is that discourses of nature in the new midwifery, which inform other
key sites of cultural production—its relationship to tradition, medical
technology, and space—are, paradoxically, at once foundational and
decentering; these discourses are part of a cultural process that works
to instill a set of gender expectations within the vocation of midwifery as well as within the experiences of pregnancy and childbirth.

First, I make what might seem the obvious argument that the new
midwifery in Canada challenges the powerful discourses of science
and medicine which have so far shaped women's embodied subjectivity. Specifically, midwifery promotes gender expectations of birthing women as strong and capable—counteracting versions of birthing
women as incapable and weak, and of birth as some thing that *happens to* women, rather than as something that women *do*. Further, I
argue that the rhetorically powerful and apparently familiar notion
of birth as a natural phenomenon—the opposite of biomedicine and
its relations of social control—is being redefined and relived by the
pragmatic choices of women in ways that reflect and promote a fundamental shift away from fixed or essentialized understandings of the
body, birth, and gender. It is a version of nature that makes room for

biomedical treatments and technologies, underpinned by the logics of caring and choice. In so doing, midwifery in Ontario works to replace current cultural versions of the pregnant and birthing body with better—but equally cultural—ones. For, as Marilyn Strathern has said, "Nature cannot survive without cultural intervention" (1992,174). Thus, new expectations of spatial and embodied experiences in pregnancy and birth give rise to deeply personal yet highly political gendered performances that are *naturalized* in the body.[4]

My study is appropriately set in the temporal and cultural context of what Emily Martin has described as "the end of the body" (1992,121) or what religious studies scholar Pamela Klassen has called the transition to "post-biomedical bodies" (2001)—a space between medicalization and resistance. The medicalization of childbirth lies, of course, in the deep cross currents of Enlightenment thinking (with its focus on the mastery of nature), the history of industrialization and the rationalization of work and everyday life, the rise of specialization in medicine, and, finally, the dichotomization of gender norms.[5] Yet, even as we acknowledge medicalization as absolutely key to understanding contemporary childbirth and the movements to reform and resist it, we must also remember that biomedicine is not monolithic. Many physicians themselves were sympathetic to midwifery before it became legalized, and some even provided backup services to midwives in the community. A great many more physicians have now welcomed midwifery into the system. Many hospitals now have birthing suites complete with baths and birthing stools and even ballet bars for upright births; midwives work in hospitals too, "among the machines" (De Vries 1997), attending more than half their clients in this setting.

In this context, the new midwifery in Canada is a venue for negotiating the medical knowledge, routines, and technologies currently in place for the cultural and clinical management of pregnancy and birth. More profoundly, it offers a reconceptualization of bodies and spaces, using nature as its guiding metaphor. Nature in midwifery is an ideal wherein choice is paramount, interventions are negotiable, and trust characterizes the midwife-client relationship. Thus, we see midwifery not solely in terms of "the romance of resistance" (to borrow Abu-

Lughod's [1990a] phrase) against a demonized biomedical system but also in terms of "discipline and dissent" (Lock and Scheper-Hughes 1990). Ultimately, in this study of contemporary midwifery in Ontario, we see that what is at stake is nothing less than "the cultural negotiation of gender in a world shaped by both social diversity and scientific hegemony" (Rapp 1991, 392).

Some Notes on Methods

This project began with fourteen months of fieldwork with midwives and their clients in the province of Ontario in 1996 and 1997. My methods involved participant observation at midwifery clinics, prenatal classes, professional meetings, and midwifery-attended home births, as well as fifty-one formal interviews with midwives and clients. My early fieldnotes were filled with descriptions of bucolic rural scenes evoking a sense of traveling and difference. For example, after speaking to Karina several times on the phone, she invited me to come and spend some time at her midwifery clinic in rural southern Ontario. Karina is a British-trained nurse midwife, who after years of working overseas, returned to practice nursing and community midwifery in her home town in Ontario in the early 1980s. When I asked for the address of her clinic, she replied, "How should I know? I just know how to get there." I set out late, in the rain, without a map, just with Karina's directions of side roads and landmarks in my head. I ended up in a small town and pulled up to the general store. I went inside to ask directions, but there was no one in sight. I called out several times and waited. Still no one appeared. I found a map of the region and left four dollars on the counter. On the road I passed lines of children waiting for the school bus and horse-drawn buggies with bright orange signs—*Slow Moving Vehicle*—that spit gravel on the shoulders. I passed miles of well-kept Mennonite farms with signs at the end of long lanes: *Maple syrup. Summer sausage. No Sunday sales.*

My destination was a small village with one main street. The sign into the village said the bridge was out and gave directions for a detour. I found the clinic in a business plaza on the outskirts of the village next to an insurance agent and a real estate office. The waiting room was full of the kind of chairs you might find in a doctor's office and a couple of rocking chairs with quilted cushions. Bookcases lined two walls, and a corner was devoted to a child-sized table and chairs and a box full of books and toys. In the waiting room sat two young Mennonite women in muted print dresses and head scarves speaking in German, one pregnant and the other holding a very small baby, both beaming. I could hear voices from the back of the place, but no one came out to greet me. I need not have worried about being late. Within minutes a young woman emerged from one of the clinic rooms and came out to the waiting room to weigh her baby; the scales were in the waiting room, and after several visits I saw that weigh-ins were usually marked by a degree of fanfare and praise for big healthy babies. This young mother had cropped, bleached-blond hair, wore cut-off denim shorts, and sported two nose rings. Her baby was called Felicity. A student midwife with shaved head and a tie-dyed pantsuit showed her how to weigh the baby. Next came Karina, an older woman in a pale print dress, with her gray hair pulled back. She greeted me casually, supervised the weigh-in, and then turned to greet the two young Mennonite women. The three of them disappeared down the hall. The office administrator put me to work stuffing envelopes, answering phones, making tea, greeting clients, and sending them in for appointments. I stayed until late afternoon and drove home in the rain.

The idea of the field of midwifery in Ontario as "distant other" may be lent some legitimacy by its history of erasure and suppression and, more recently, by its existence as a grassroots countercultural movement located on the margins of mainstream society and maternity care. Ethnographic fieldwork at the turn of the twenty-first century, however, does not necessarily require a journey over land, or sea, or political borders. Nor does it demand a novel or exotic subject. Being in the field is more a matter of looking and listening in particular anthropological ways, rather than being in particular kinds of anthropological places. Indeed, the difficult task of conducting fieldwork "at home" is that rather than making the subject appear other, one must make the familiar within it explicit.

My experience of doing fieldwork at home was marked by a particular set of methodological dislocations that inevitably became part of the production of knowledge. I was studying midwifery in a time of tremendous change, and I was conducting fieldwork at home in a discipline historically committed to studies of social, geographical, and cultural others. Initially, for example, I found it quite difficult to even get to the field. Midwives are extremely busy people. In the years following incorporation, most sat on multiple committees setting up the new Midwifery Education Program and the new College of Midwives, while running their clinical practices and trying to maintain their personal lives. I often spent time in a field occupied not by bodies but by telephones, faxes, electronic messages, appointment books, cars, and crowded streetcars. I seemed to spend a lot of time waiting. I went to interview appointments many times to find midwives had been called away to precipitous births, had stayed two days at a long labor, or three days at back-to-back labors, or had simply gone home to sleep. These experiences—which might have been counted as failures—nevertheless became part of my knowledge of midwifery.

Another important methodological note to mention is the move in feminist social science toward developing collaborative relationships in the field and also toward openly situating ourselves personally and politically.[6] I have described myself elsewhere as an "interested researcher" of midwifery—someone with a long history of research and activism in women's reproductive health who is also an anthropologist committed to critical reflection and analysis (MacDonald and Bourgeault 2002). My personal, political, and scholarly intentions are entwined by a feminist epistemology that holds that research can facilitate the disclosure of social processes that construct and organize knowledge that shapes the everyday lives of women (Stanley and Wise 1990). Despite the challenges of getting to the field, my position as an interested researcher ultimately helped me develop rapport with midwives and their clients. Though I was not, for the most part, explicit about my political opinions, midwives and women in my study assumed (correctly) that I was supportive of professional midwifery, and this no doubt eased my entry.

This was not uniformly the case, however, and I was reminded on several occasions that I was very much an outsider. One midwifery practice that I approached declined to participate in my study, saying they did not consider it a worthwhile use of their time. Another practice where I had done several months of volunteer work and participant observation informed me out of the blue one day that my time was up. (The staff had decided at a practice meeting the week before that the clinic was too crowded with clients, midwives, and midwifery students to have another body around.)

Typically, I was carefully screened by midwives on the basis of my specific interests as a researcher. What did I want to know? What would I write or say about midwifery? My growing awareness of the controversies within the midwifery community in the post-legislation years found me, at later stages in the research process, prefacing my requests for interviews with statements like: "My research is not about the process of the professionalization of midwifery." Even so, I vividly recall an exchange with a midwife I hoped to interview in which I was told, "If you are interested in describing how legalizing midwifery destroyed the dream of an independent midwifery in Ontario then I will not speak to you." As Visweswaran (1994) notes, the close and idealized egalitarian relations that some feminists envision between researcher and researched can be elusive and are sometimes illusory. Individual women, too, exercised their choice to speak to me or not. One of my first conversations at an urban midwifery practice where I conducted participant observation was with a Muslim woman who talked excitedly to me about her faith, her first pregnancy, and the wonderful care of midwives. Although she told me she thought my work was important and wished me luck, she firmly declined to be interviewed formally.

Midwives and Clients

Over the course of my fieldwork I conducted participant observation in five different clinics. I made intensive one-week visits at two clinics, and spent one or two days a week at three other clinics over the course of three, four, and six months, respectively. By the end of my fourteen months in the field, I had conducted twenty-six interviews with midwives and twenty-five with midwifery clients. I have begun to draw a picture of community midwives as a group of well-educated, motivated, even tireless, women dedicated to a set of clinical practices embedded in a larger ideological agenda and moving toward social change. Most midwives in Ontario in the late 1990s were white, middle class, and well educated, either by formal means or self-taught. Ethnic and linguistic diversity in the profession has increased in the past decade, as the education program reaches out to draw in students from diverse communities and the College of Midwives refines its procedures for registering midwives trained in other jurisdictions.

The midwives in my study varied in age from mid-twenties to mid-sixties, and varied too in terms of marital status, sexual orientation, motherhood, and geographical location across the province, with some of the concerns of rural and northern midwives being much different than southern and urban midwives. The clinics I volunteered in were full of activity and opportunities for conversation with both midwives and clients. The formal interviews I conducted with midwives were set apart from clinic routines and spaces, and were often conducted in cafes, restaurants, or midwives' homes. The interviews were semistructured and open-ended, designed to elicit what I call midwifery narratives—stories of becoming and being a midwife.

Like midwives, women who sought midwifery care in Ontario in the late 1990s also tended to be white, middle class, and relatively well educated, most having had some postsecondary education. They, too, have slowly diversified in terms of cultural, linguistic, and socioeconomic background, especially as midwives themselves diversify and the outreach programs at many clinics draw in new immigrants and ethnic communities. Most of the women I interviewed formally were either married or in long-term relationships with men; one was single, and two had female partners. Many worked outside the home as social workers, students, lawyers, civil servants, teachers, and nurses. Others worked in their homes as artists or writers.[7]

Midwives tend to call the women to whom they provide care "midwifery clients," though I have sometimes heard them called by more intimate terms such as "my ladies," "my mothers," or "my women." In the social and institutional realms beyond the clinic, however, or when referred to collectively, they are more often referred to as "midwifery consumers." The idea of the midwifery consumer remains important because it speaks to the consumer-based campaigns for choices in childbirth that were fundamental to the success of midwifery as a social movement in Canada.[8] The idea of the midwifery consumer also speaks to issues of class, especially as understood by sociologist Daniel Miller. Regardless of income, Miller notes, members of the middle class develop themselves as consumers with tastes that express something about them—their education, politics, feminist sensibilities, autonomy, environmental politics—what Miller calls "skills of consumption" (1997, 71). Choosing to consume midwifery services is not quite so simple an expression of class as it appears, when all maternity services are equally covered in the public Ontario Health Insurance Plan (OHIP) and when the gold standard of maternity care in Canada has been the specialist care of an obstetrician, even for normal birth. Consuming midwifery then is a very particular kind of expression of an "alternative" taste, and many women told me it often came at some personal cost. Indeed, the vast majority of the women in my study had been subject to the unsolicited scrutiny and even condemnation of family, friends, physicians, co-workers, and strangers for their choice to use midwives. Such expressions of opposition to midwifery, however, simultaneously mark its distinctiveness and value as an alternative.

As with the midwife interviews, the client interviews were semistructured and open-ended. Most of the midwifery clients I interviewed were drawn from the clinics in which I conducted participant observation, though several contacted me independently, having heard of my work through the grapevine. All interviews took place at their homes, which were the most convenient and comfortable locations for women with infants and small children. In several instances, women's partners were present for all of the interview or intermittently throughout, adding important details and provoking interesting exchanges. Most of the interviews lasted between one-and-a-half and three hours, but I often spent much longer with women and their families, drinking tea, holding babies, viewing birth videos and photo albums, touring upstairs rooms and gardens. The client interviews were designed to elicit another kind of midwifery narrative—stories of pregnancy and birth with midwifery care.

It was clear to me from the beginning that my study participants were active cultural producers (Ong 1995) and indeed sophisticated political strategists, who played a part in shaping the research for this book. Most of them were interested in engaging in the theoretical questions central to my study, whether they approached the question from personal experience or a broader political agenda. Women who had midwifery care, acting on their own interpretation of what I wanted to know, gave long glowing reports about the caring, knowledgeable, and tireless midwives who attended them. They gave articulate political speeches against the medicalization of birth and shared intimate details about their personal relationships with parents, partners, and siblings. Midwives, too, used my interviews to reiterate arguments about women's choice, recount their personal trials working within the profession, air their views on controversial issues, or tell me what they thought I should know about midwifery and nothing more. Ethnographic subjects exercise power; they refuse, deny, omit, redirect, insist, opine. It was in many ways an experience of "studying up" or, at the very least, across.

A Field of Narratives

Medical anthropologists have long employed the elicitation of narratives of health, illness, and healing as a methodological strategy (DiGiacomo 1987; Kleinman 1988; MacDonald 1994).[9] The move toward valuing individual narratives in qualitative research is one of the ways that medical anthropologists continue to challenge the impoverished clinical gaze of biomedicine. Listening to women's birth narratives, as a methodology, was, for my purposes, as important as being there to witness or to "verify" "actual" events. Anthropologist Mitra Emad offers a compelling way to conceptualize the study of discursive constructions and performances of the body. In her study of acupuncture clients in the United States, Emad focuses on what she calls "stories of emergent bodies," whereby individuals understand their bodies and selves to have been transformed in some way, through the experience of acupuncture and its "disclosure" (1996, 2). She describes this as an "embodied way of demarcating the field" within the wider field of American society that is not necessarily spatially nor temporally specific—an approach that I find fits well with my own field and my own research task.

The midwifery narratives told to me by clients were intensely personal, individually meaningful, and often personally transformative. Yet, even in the most personal stories, there may be a sense of "worldliness." The women who spoke to me were aware of midwifery's structurally marginal past and socially vulnerable present. Most had a sense of participating in the larger collective struggle taking place within Ontario and beyond by choosing midwifery and also by participating in my study. Some had been politically active in the midwifery or home birth movements prior to regulation. Telling a personal story that is politically motivated transgresses the boundary between private and public by bringing the everyday details of private life into the public domain (Salazar 1991). At the same time, most women in my study described themselves as average women wanting what was best for themselves and their babies. Again, it is in precisely this sense that these women understood themselves to be politically motivated in choosing midwifery care and in choosing to tell their stories to me: they want their personal stories to be documented to serve as counterstories to the institutionalization and medicalization of birth. They want their stories to emerge from the margins to take their place in the public domain of knowledge about "normal" pregnancy and childbirth.

Midwifery and the Politics of Representation

Although part of my experience of the field was trying to get to it, when the work was done, I could not seem to leave it. Not only do I run into my former "informants" in restaurants and grocery stores, I regularly see midwives at conferences and academic talks on midwifery or health—including those given by me about them. It seems that my interpretations and representations of midwifery are never far from scrutiny, and it has been impossible for me to establish my privilege and authority to speak about midwifery on the basis of having come away from a distant field, back to the academy, armed with knowledge and the power to speak it. (Though this has never been my goal.) The politics of representation have often loomed large over the course of my fieldwork and writing on midwifery. I consider my work a midwifery narrative of another sort—a critical scholarly interpretation that takes its place in a broader field of midwifery descriptions and debates.

Since midwifery was declared a profession in the province of Ontario, the efforts of scholars, midwives, advocates, and critics to represent midwifery—to say what it is at the moment of its transformation—have intensified. Sociological and historical accounts have begun to appear. The popular media has offered both high praise and profound skepticism.[10] Politically active, working midwives, meanwhile, lament the fact that they have no time to tell the story themselves. The struggle to represent midwifery in Canada at this critical juncture is important because of the prominence that community midwifery holds in the broader movements across North America advocating for women's health and childbirth reform. In short, community midwifery has become the symbol *par excellence* of women wresting control over reproduction from a patriarchal biomedical system (Bourgeault 2006). Read this way, the story of midwifery's reemergence and legitimation in Canada is a story of triumph. Indeed, many have lauded the Ontario midwifery model of care as maintaining key aspects of the social movement—including the hard-won allowance for home birth—while gaining legitimacy in the public eye, not to mention public funding. Others, however, feel that with professionalization has come co-optation and the end of a truly independent midwifery in which midwives offered real choice to Ontario women away from the watchful eye of the state. Meanwhile, the road to regulation and the actual process of incorporation into a health care system that sometimes received these new professionals with hostility was bumpy, to say the least. (See Chapter 2.) Some community midwives had no desire to join the mainstream system, while others found themselves fighting against the exclusionary practices of the new profession.

The immediacy of midwives' concerns over the representation of their new profession by outsiders are certainly warranted; some midwives fear that midwifery will be misrepresented in social science research, and some suggested my authority to represent midwifery was limited by my outsider status. It is important to mention this from the outset because the tricky politics of representation have been part of the social context of midwifery in Ontario from the moment I began this work and remain salient even as I write. Taking a broader view, one of the main thrusts of feminist social science research and writing on midwifery and childbirth has been to make women's lives and knowledge and work more visible. Anthropologists studying pregnancy and birth in non-Western settings, for example, have typically sought to validate traditional or indigenous midwives by revealing the cultural and clinical logic of their beliefs and practices (Jordan 1993, 1978; Laderman 1983; MacCormack 1982; McClain 1989; Sargent 1989). Anthropologists studying pregnancy and birth in Western settings have also sought to validate the embodied experiences of pregnant and birthing women (Davis-Floyd 1992; Klassen 2001) and the knowledge of the women who attend them (Davis-Floyd and Davis 1997; Fraser 1995). At the same time, feminist ethnographers have been concerned with issues of responsibility and accountability to the groups and individuals with whom they work, as well as with the social consequences for women who speak to them and the political consequences of their work (Stacey 1991).

How might a feminist ethnographer represent other women without betraying their interests (Ong 1995)? How can one balance critical exegesis with authorial responsibility? Midwives, while giving of their time in the interests of the goal of visibility for their profession and its social project, are aware of their ongoing vulnerability and wary of critical interpretations. Could my description and interpretation of midwifery in Ontario, while making midwifery more visible, also expose its vulnerabilities? Could something that I write— an intimate description of home birth or an airing of the differences within this nascent profession—be used in some way to discredit midwifery? The controversial allowance for home birth is particularly vulnerable to scrutiny and attack, and midwifery in Ontario continues to be watched closely by both supporters and detractors in other provinces. For example, an article appearing in the *Society of Obstetricians and Gynaecologists of Canada Journal* attacked home birth as "a dangerous, inappropriate and irrelevant" part of midwifery and disparages "midwifery advocates who constitute the militant wing of this movement (who) have exalted home birth and linked it utterly with the idea of professional midwifery" (Goodwin 1997, 1181).[11] To more fully address the politics of representation in midwifery at this time, I turn now to some of the keys issues that came to light in the process of professionalization itself.

Shadow Stories

> Fieldnote entry, April 15, 1997: Interview with midwife, Lillian. *Shades of Fictions of Feminist Ethnography.* She evaded several of my questions, especially the ones about the inquest [into an infant death] and also about the pros and cons of regulation. In order to—what?—to smooth it over? To tell the tale of a good outcome? Or perhaps to say "mind your own business."

I conducted this research in the wake of midwifery professionalization and the publication of a number of scholarly descriptions of midwifery in Canada, including several in Ontario which were received by midwives as particularly critical. In the most painfully controversial critique, sociologist Sheryl Nestel argues that the incorporation of midwifery in Ontario was a racist process that systematically excluded hundreds of foreign-trained and immigrant women of color in order to preserve midwifery as "a new profession for the white middle classes" (1996). Some in the midwifery community rejected the charge of racism as harsh and inaccurate. Others accepted the criticism in part but argued that it was premature. They pointed to the work that has been done since legislation to formally acknowledge the credentials of women trained in other jurisdictions, and to reach out to different cultural communities in the recruitment of midwifery students. Initially, a very few midwives welcomed Nestel's observations as part of open and ongoing dialogue between midwifery and the communities it serves and overlaps.

Another issue dates back to the late 1980s and concerns the contest from within community midwifery itself over whether to pursue professionalization at all. Jutta Mason, a long-time midwifery supporter and critic of professionalization in Ontario warned in an essay, "The Trouble with Licensing Midwives" (1990), that the regulation of midwifery in Ontario would draw women back into a system of knowledge and authority they had deliberately opted out of and would ultimately reduce women's choices in childbirth by circumscribing midwives' autonomy. Mason predicted that midwives would be used to watch over and discipline women—in the Foucauldian sense—on behalf of biomedicine and the state. A recent example of the kind of surveillance that Mason fears is illustrated in the "Healthy Babies, Healthy Children" initiative by the Ontario provincial government in which all maternity care providers are being asked to administer a questionnaire to new mothers in order to determine those who are "at risk" and in need of follow-up by a social service agency. It is a well-intentioned program, perhaps, but one that uses midwives to draw women into a system where they may be labeled and subjected to intervention by the state. Many midwives are uneasy about taking part in such programs. Mason also noted that with professionalization, non-registered midwives and birthing women would face criminal prosecution if they tried to opt out of the system in order to avoid the gaze of biomedicine and the state. Finally, sociologist Ivy Bourgeault's critique focused on the erosion of the close relationship between midwife and client—a hallmark of client-centered community midwifery outside the system—created by professionalization (2006).

My purpose here is not to debate these specific charges but to consider some of the effects of such scholarly critiques on professional midwifery at what must still be considered a vulnerable time. Certainly, these critiques call our attention to differences among midwives and their community of clients, supporters, and chroniclers—including myself—about what is *good* for midwifery. Certainly, it may be argued that community midwifery in Ontario in many ways thrived in a state of subversive and resistant marginality of its own choosing.

Indeed, many midwives and women wish it had never been incorpo-rated into the system at all. On the other hand, professional midwifery may be capable of mounting an arguably greater (faster? more visible? broader?) challenge to the prevailing cultural system of medicalized birth than a midwifery in the margins. This was a gamble that most midwives and midwifery consumers in the province were willing to take when the question of incorporation was pressed upon them. The story of the incorporation of midwifery in Ontario is, of course, mul-tilayered. There are many examples of what Jo Anne Myers–Cieko calls the "shadow stories" of regulating independent or community midwifery in Canada and the United States (1997 personal communi-cation).[12] Among the shadow stories in Ontario are the experiences of those within the midwifery community who opposed professionaliza-tion; radical midwives with many years of experience in the move-ment suffered from the disciplinary power of the new regulated sys-tem. Many other experienced midwives who were not admitted to the Michener Pre-registration Program lost their livelihoods the in-stant midwifery was declared a profession, including long-time ru-ral midwives without sufficient numbers of births per year to qualify for pre-registration.[13] When these rural midwives ceased to practice, many rural women were left without midwives in their communi-ties.[14] One of the saddest shadow stories of the incorporation of mid-wifery in Ontario was the death of an infant at a midwife-attended home birth in the rural community of Durham in 1990, on the eve of regulation. The public inquest that followed was not only devastating for those personally involved but also threatened to cast a shadow over all of midwifery in terms of its acceptance in the public eye.

When I began this study, both the shadow and the success stories surfaced quickly and with passion. Finding the balance between such losses and gains is perhaps the challenge for midwifery itself as it con-tinues to take shape and grow in Ontario. While this book is not pri-marily about the process of professionalization or its shadow stories, my focus does not ignore the lingering wounds and questions of this era, nor the new issues brought to bear on midwifery by its current context within the health care and education systems. If this work has a public intellectual goal, it is a rather cultural one: to bring to light new stories to serve as counterpoints to hegemonic biomedical stories about pregnancy, birth, and birth attendance, and also to illuminate midwifery as a dynamic and necessarily contested, cultural system. Bringing new stories to light was often the explicit reason women gave for wanting to tell me their stories. Fittingly, telling and listening to stories is part of the clinical work of midwifery itself—part of the work of creating a sense of shared knowledge and responsibility. This clinical metaphor may be the most apt for describing the contribution of this particular anthropological story about midwifery in Canada; it is part of the shared knowledge and responsibility with others writing and acting about midwifery from other positions and places. Such interpretive intersections may be fraught, but they are also productive. The perspectival partiality of truth inherent in stories of all kinds—personal, professional, and academic—is one of the most compelling claims of postcolonial ethnography and feminist critiques of objectivity, and it is what I offer in this book.

CHAPTER TWO

Tales of Loss and Renaissance

T HE HISTORY OF MIDWIFERY in Canada has often been read as a tale of loss and endurance in which the traditional, women-centered, home-based midwifery birth culture of the eighteenth and nineteenth centuries was stamped out by the rising medical profession and the march of progress. I continue with a more nuanced history below, but it is important to see how this particular version might serve as an important point of reference for contemporary midwifery—an origin story of sorts—informing its unique social meaning and clinical approach. I address the uses of history (and imagined histories) in the contemporary project of building midwifery identity in Chapter 3, but here I begin the history of midwifery in Canada with a more conventional approach, tracing the processes involved in the near demise of traditional forms of midwifery, the emergence of midwifery as a social movement in the 1970s and 1980s, its transformation into a movement for professionalization, and the process by which it was incorporated into the health system in Ontario in the 1990s. Finally, I outline the current mechanisms of public funding, education, licensure, and access to midwifery as a profession and for clients seeking midwifery care.

Historical Forms of Midwifery in Canada

Historical forms of midwifery varied considerably across Canada in the eighteenth and nineteenth centuries. Neighbor networks of empirical midwives were common in Ontario and the West, while in parts of Nova Scotia, Quebec, and Newfoundland professional midwives were trained and appointed by either the Church or the Crown. To varying degrees, professional and empirical midwives transported their knowledge and skills from intact traditions in Europe, while Aboriginal midwives served their communities as they had done for generations (Benoit 1991; Biggs 1983; Laforce 1990; Kaufert and O'Neil 1993; Mason 1987; Mitchenson 2002).[1]

Neighbor networks of empirical midwives were the most common form of midwifery in Ontario, and the majority of women were assisted in childbirth by middle-aged and older women, respected in their communities, who, having given birth themselves, were called upon for their expertise. Their clinical knowledge was gained informally or through apprenticeship. In addition to clinical support, the social and material aspects of birth attendance were very important; along with other women in the community, midwives provided gifts of food and clothing, as well as housework and childcare for the women they attended. Their clinical work began with labor and continued through to postpartum care for the mother, breastfeeding support, and newborn care. Especially in rural settings, midwifery did not exist as a profession in the sense that there were probably few women whose primary work was that of attending women in childbirth; most women who acted as midwives to their neighbors and relatives also raised children and were engaged in the productive labor of the household, such as farm work (Mason 1987).

It is important to emphasize the plurality of forms rather than rely on the universalizing trope of "traditional midwifery" for which the neighbor midwife has tended to serve as the dominant motif in both scholarly and popular histories. As historian Lesley Biggs points out, the idea of a singular midwifery tradition in Canada "homogenises a range of birth attendants under one rubric" (2004, 22), eliding other forms, whereas midwifery in Canada was more varied and its demise more uneven. The fall of traditional midwifery writ large has nevertheless figured prominently in popular and scholarly feminist analyses of midwifery in Canada (Barrington 1985; James-Chetalet 1989; Mason 1987; Shroff 1998) and also appears in midwives' own narratives about their historical antecedents—although sometimes in critical ways (MacDonald 2004). The rhetorical uses to which the icon of traditional midwifery has been put in the social and professional projects of contemporary midwifery is an important topic that I take up in Chapter 3.

Some historical accounts of midwifery in North America—particularly those referring to black and Aboriginal women—describe midwifery as a sacred calling (Dougherty 1978; Hoch-Smith and Spring 1978; Susie 1988). In contrast, historical accounts of midwifery among European settlers and their descendents tend to characterize it more as a set of everyday practices, a gendered social role embedded in women's domestic culture, rather than as highly specialized knowledge or ritual.[2]

As Mason describes,

So the baby was born and the bread was done. Having a baby, while it was seen as a very special occasion, did not involve a radical break from the business of everyday life . . . The event of birth was so securely entwined with the other work of women—the preparation of food, the manufacturing of clothing, the maintaining of the home . . . The birthing woman was surrounded by other women she knew who shared her life and fate and status in most respects (1987, 202–3).

Though laws restricting the practice of midwifery were enacted as early as 1795, they were often not enforced (Biggs 1983). They likely served, however, to intimidate women who attended each other's births and to discourage women from organizing themselves so as to make midwifery a profession (Connor 1994 in Bourgeault 2006, 45). Lack of organization among neighbor midwives was almost certainly underpinned by the numerous demands that these midwives already had on their time as wives, mothers, and farm workers (Bourgeault 2006). Barriers of language and geography in rural settlements must have contributed as well.

The latter half of the nineteenth century marked the beginning of the decline of most forms of midwifery in Canada and, indeed, throughout North America. The key factor in this process was arguably the expansion of biomedicine and the rise of medical specialization. Physicians, fighting to secure their professional niches, waged a successful campaign to discredit midwives as a group, claiming they were dirty, ignorant, and incompetent (Ehrenreich and English 1973; Mason 1987; Mitchenson 2002; Sullivan and Weitz 1988; Rushing 1988). The empirical neighbor midwife was particularly vulnerable to attack. Integral to the displacement of midwifery was the redefinition of childbirth as a medical event, fraught with danger, and in need of intervention by obstetricians. The growing cultural authority of obstetrical medicine was reinforced by the growing authority of science more generally; it was not necessarily based on the demonstration of better maternal and infant outcomes—indeed, the opposite was true. As Mason (1987) points out, mortality statistics in hospitals were higher than births in the community at this time. Thus the rise of the predominantly male profession over the predominantly female one must be seen in part as a political battle, in which the right to a medical monopoly over childbearing was "the prize" (Jezioranski 1987, 95).

Another important historical factor in the demise of traditional forms of midwifery was the Industrial Revolution, which was influential in redefining birth as a medical-mechanical event (Davis-Floyd 1994; Martin 1987; Susie 1988). While physicians filled the roles of the managers of the mechanical process of birth, the midwife, in contrast, was more like a craftsperson. "The time she took to perform her craft was unfashionably slow and long, as was the natural course of labor and delivery. The hospital, on the other hand, employed technology to "speed up" and make painless the birth process; it was modeled after the modern factory—efficient assembly line care with a rigid schedule" (Susie 1988, 3). In addition, gender ideals of women as frail and dependent—and therefore incapable of either giving or attending birth unaided by male experts—flourished during this time, especially among the middle and upper classes (James-Chetalet 1989; Mitchenson 1991). Thus, "women's perceptions of themselves influenced their choice of birth attendants and the resulting system of maternity care" (James-Chetalet 1989, 421).[3]

The increase in physician-attended births did have its critics at the time; the management of birth by male obstetricians, some objected, threatened female modesty. Others pointed out that obstetric practice lacked scientific support (Biggs 1983). Many communities opposed the policies that curtailed midwifery and continued to call on their local midwives out of loyalty and, due to physician shortages across the country, necessity.[4] Nevertheless, obstetric ideology and practice radiated steadily outward from urban centers, and by the 1940s midwifery was no longer a maternity care option for the vast majority of Canadian women (James-Chetalet 1989, 268). Traditional forms of midwifery were retained in some Mennonite, Hutterite, and First Nations communities, as well as in rural and remote areas (Benoit 1991; Biggs 1983; Campanella et al. 1993; Plummer 2000.). For example, midwifery in Newfoundland and Labrador continued because of that province's late entry into Confederation in 1948, its stronger ties to Britain (where nurse-midwifery was part of the health care system), and the extreme remoteness of many out-port communities (Benoit 1991). Meanwhile, British trained nurse-midwives were hired to manage births in nursing stations in the far North from the late 1950s until the 1970s when an official policy of evacuation to southern hospitals for all pregnant Aboriginal women was enforced (Kaufert and O'Neil 1993; Plummer 2000). Ironically, this policy was implemented in Aboriginal communities at the same time that midwifery and home birth was gaining popularity and moving towards state acceptance in the south (Kaufert and O'Neil 1993; O'Neil and Kaufert 1990).

Community Midwifery in Ontario

What has been dubbed in scholarly circles "the new midwifery" in Canada grew out of sweeping social changes in the 1960s and 1970s. It grew in response to women seeking more "natural," family-centered, and fulfilling birth experiences (Barrington 1985). Consumer advocates for natural childbirth since the 1970s and the failure of the natural childbirth movement to move beyond co-optation by the medical establishment further encouraged interest in midwifery in North America (Van Wagner 1991). The home birth movement was especially influential.[5] Proponents of the midwifery movement saw birth as a natural, rather than medical event, and advocated the reallocation of responsibility for pregnancy and birth from physicians to parents, and the relocation of birth from the hospital to the home. Ideologically, the purpose of midwifery as a social movement was also to reinvent positive gender roles for women. Thus, to the discourse of nature and tradition was added the liberal feminist rhetoric of choice, rights, and health—reflecting diverse political alliances (Rushing 1993). The strength of midwifery as a social movement was bolstered by strategic links to the women's health movement, which pursued greater control and choice for women in all reproductive health matters. Scholars and women's health activists identified the birth process as a site of women's oppression and therefore a focus for emancipation (Arms 1975; Corea 1985; Oakley 1984; O'Brien 1981; Rothman 1982). Midwifery was not just on the radical feminist agenda, however. Middle-class notions about togetherness in marriage and the exaltation of motherhood—in both alternative and conservative strains—contributed as well (Michaelson 1988, 4). A rash of physician-authored books criticizing medicalization and advocating educated alternatives also fueled the fire, drawing not so much on the rhetoric of female empowerment as on the imagery of women's true nature.[6]

The (re)emergence of midwifery in North America in the popular and scholarly imagination is a tale of renaissance and the restoration of its "historical beginnings"—a birth culture characterized by strong ties between women, sound empirical knowledge about birth, a central role and status for midwives, and more individual choice and personal control for birthing women. Indeed, the fall and rise of midwifery in Canada and elsewhere came to typify the struggle of women against the patriarchal medical establishment, against prevailing conceptions of birth as pathological, and against outworn notions of women as incapable and weak. The tendency to essentialize women and universalize birth in this formulation was a strategic aspect of sophisticated critiques of medicalized and institutionalized birth in the West. Thus, the rise of community midwifery in Canada was predicated in part—and effectively so—on "the dissension of other things" (Foucault 1984, 79).

By the mid-1980s an estimated fifty midwives had established practices in Ontario and were providing care to about 1,500 birthing women a year (Van Wagner 1988, 115; Tyson 1991). *Community midwifery* was a name that those involved took on themselves to replace the term *lay midwifery* to describe birth attendance conducted outside the health care system. The term also emphasized the decentralized nature of childbirth attendance and the close relationship between the community midwife and her constituents (Burtch 1988, 354).[7] Van Wagner also notes the strong links between community midwifery and shifts in public health thinking and policy towards a "community health" model that takes social, economic, environmental, and political conditions into account, focuses on health promotion, and shows concern for equity and access to care (1991, 74). The essence of this new midwifery was not to create another childbirth authority but to put control of the process back in the hands of the women giving birth. Thus midwifery during this time was consumer driven and regulated, and women's experience ideally determined midwifery knowledge and practice.

Community midwifery training in Ontario was eclectic. Most women began slowly by simply attending one another's births at home. Then they developed their skills over a number of years through some combination of self-teaching, participation in study groups, formal course work from accredited midwifery programs in the United States or the United Kingdom, and apprenticeship with more experienced or foreign-trained nurse-midwives. Few midwives in Ontario are solely apprentice trained. Many more combined self-teaching and apprenticeships with short-term intensive training at privately run midwifery clinics in El Paso, Texas, and Jamaica.[8] Overall, the ideals of apprenticeship training—to learn by watching and doing—were held in high esteem.

The way Isobel became a midwife is typical of many in the province, combining personal experience, training in the community, and formal training. She began attending births in the mid-1970s after giving birth at home, attended by a sympathetic local physician. She studied with other women in her community and was invited regularly to home births. Isobel was surprised when, after a time, she heard someone refer to her as a midwife. Eventually, she entered a nursing program and earned her diploma. She then went to work in a local hospital, earning a reputation for her knowledge about labor, birth, and lactation. She continued to attend home births and remained committed to the midwifery movement in Ontario. Isobel's experience illustrates the ambivalence many community midwives felt with regard to their own education and training before regulation.

> I didn't feel like a midwife until I had acquired a certain experience, knowledge, and skill. For me that was always important. So I couldn't quite accept that a midwife was a midwife only because her community calls her that.

While in favor of formal training for herself, Isobel thinks there are other valid routes of gaining competence as a midwife.

> The whole idea of a protected title—that exclusivity didn't appeal to me either. What I wanted to do was honor women who were acting as midwives, women that were attending births, or women that were doing that kind of work—labor coaches (which is an awful term) and doulas, or postpartum support workers, or pregnancy counselors, or La Leche League, or childbirth educators—all those people were doing a similar kind of work. But I really—I do believe that you have to have some knowledge and skills to have the title of midwife. Now what those are— there's some varying ideas about what core competency should be. You know, how many catches do you have to have? Or what skills do you have to have? Are you a midwife if you can't fit a diaphragm or do a pap test? . . . I think that women—especially in rural areas who are maybe the only women around who can help a woman have the birth she wants to have—I think more power to them. But I really worry too because I've seen some things that are scary and seen midwives give advice to women that I think is dangerous to them. But, then again, it's the same thing that doctors and nurses can do in their so-called profession.

Barrington (1985) and Bourgeault (2006, 91–92) suggest that it is inaccurate to view midwifery at this time as unregulated. Midwives earned the respect of the community; thus, they were accredited by parents rather than the state. As the prospect of state regulation grew closer in Ontario however, matters of training, experience, and scope of practice, which had previously been more flexible and varied by region, became more contested. On the one hand, legal recognition of midwifery by the province would validate the skills and experience community midwives had worked so hard to acquire outside the system. On the other hand, it would involve a process of exclusion: legitimation within the system for some, and loss of status and livelihood for others. Many midwives in the province were for regulation but felt ambivalent about the exclusion that formal education and training would entail.

Not surprisingly, the expansion of midwifery in the 1970s and early 1980s also sparked concern among physicians about competition and safety. Some midwives had learned their skills by attending births at home and in hospital as labor coaches with sympathetic physicians. These "home birth doctors," though few in number, contributed significantly to the education of midwives in Ontario and to the support of the movement. For the most part, however, Ontario physicians did not condone or assist community midwifery prior to legislation, and they were almost unanimous in their opposition to home birth. Their knowledge of community midwifery came from the upsetting occasions when midwifery clients or newborns were brought from home to hospital—sometimes in an ambulance. Hospital personnel generally did not recognize such transports as appropriate care but rather saw them as "midwifery disasters" and "botched home births." Few physicians or nurses at this time would have had any knowledge of all the midwife-attended home births that occurred without incident. Women transferred from midwife-attended home births were often treated with hostility, and midwives themselves were subject to prosecution for an array of charges including criminal negligence and practicing medicine without a license. Although there were few trials involving midwives in Canada, the vulnerable legal position of midwives was becoming clear.[9] Midwives in Ontario responded to this vulnerability by organizing for themselves professional associations that set formal standards of clinical practice and encouraged record keeping (Bourgeault 2006; Van Wagner 1988). The Ontario Association of Midwives (OAM) was formed in 1981; it grew out of an earlier organization, the Midwives Support and Study Group, which itself was an offshoot of the Toronto-based Home Birth Task Force. The OAM membership included birth helpers, midwives, consumers, and other midwifery supporters.

> Midwives and the women they served existed as an amorphous group with few divisions and little hierarchical separation of caregiver and client. In fact, the terms "caregiver" and "client" are not appropriate in describing the roles of each, as a far more egalitarian, friendship-oriented relationship existed than these terms connote. Often a woman would help a friend at birth and that friend would in turn help her out at childbirth. Midwives and the women they cared for were not seen as having different interests from each other. Together, they made up a small but politically active community striving for more choice and control in childbirth. (Bourgeault 1996, 69)

Bourgeault notes that the decision among midwives to seek legitimation and incorporation was largely due to "forces external to the midwifery community" (1996, 104). The first event was a high-profile coroner's inquest into the death of an infant in southwestern Ontario after a midwife-attended home birth in 1982. The inquest had the effect of rallying significant public support for midwifery. Moreover, the jury in the inquest recommended that midwifery become regulated. The inquest also motivated midwives to become more politically focused. The goal of professionalization seems to have been clarified in the wake of this inquest (Bourgeault 2006, 87). It was also at this time that the College of Physicians and Surgeons of Ontario issued a statement strongly discouraging physicians from attending home births (1982, 2). Consequently, midwives across the province who had previously practiced with physicians were forced to continue alone. Another inquest following the death of an infant on Toronto

Island in 1985 generated more publicity and controversy. The inquest into this infant death became a forum to debate public policy on midwifery and maternity care in general. This inquest, too, rallied public support and resulted in the jury's recommendation that midwifery be regulated and incorporated into the provincial health care system.

Another significant event in the move to incorporate midwifery was the establishment by the province of the Health Professions Legislation Review (HPLR) in late 1982. The HPLR contacted the OAM and the Ontario Nurse-Midwives Association (ONMA) to make submissions as to what form midwifery should take. It was strongly felt at the time that if community midwives did not make a bid for midwifery, it would be regulated anyway and they would have no input into it at all. Furthermore, the implementation of a hospital-based nurse-midwifery would have, in the words of one community midwife, "killed home birth." "The midwifery movement realized that if it did not take up the issue of regulation and seek to define its own standards of practice and training, midwives would be defined by others" (Van Wagner 1988, 116).[10]

As midwives in the province of Ontario pursued integration, they had the benefit not only of a strong social movement with a vision for a new kind of maternity care in Canada but also of knowledge of professional midwifery models that were working well—or not working well—in other jurisdictions. In shaping their vision for the new profession of midwifery in Ontario, community midwives drew on the scholarly and professional literature available on midwifery models abroad, as well as their own international networks. Some of the challenges faced by midwives in the United States, for example, were read as "cautionary tales" (Davis-Floyd 1999). It was well known that independent midwives in the United States (who worked much like community midwives in Canada prior to legislation) remained vulnerable to prosecution and were left out of the loop of third-party health insurance. American Certified Nurse Midwives, meanwhile, in some states worked without much autonomy and were restricted to hospitals only.

Some members of the OAM were also involved with the Midwifery Alliance of North America (MANA), an organization that advocates multiple routes to becoming a midwife and strives to uphold ideals and a model of practice similar to what the Ontario midwifery movement envisioned. In a show of support for the Ontario process, MANA held its 1984 annual meeting in Toronto at the same time that a Private Member's Bill arguing for the integration of midwifery was presented in the provincial legislature. Later, the provincial government-appointed Task Force on the Implementation of Midwifery in Ontario in 1986 and 1987 turned to the Netherlands, where midwifery is characterized by professional autonomy, choice of birth place, and the assumption that normal birth is the domain of midwives while abnormality is the domain of obstetricians. Low rates of intervention, high rates of patient satisfaction, and among the best infant and maternal outcome statistics in the world also recommended the Dutch model to Ontario. Thus, the model of midwifery in Ontario today is a product of local social and historical specificity and international networks and knowledge exchange.

Looking back, some in the midwifery movement clearly distinguish between midwifery as a social movement that only much later broadened its concerns to include the goal of professional and legal recognition for midwives. Others believe that the promise of legislation—a chance to be legitimate health care practitioners—was one of the key reasons that midwifery as a social movement gained momentum in the 1980s at all. In other words, they believe that midwifery as a social movement and midwifery as a professionalization movement were inseparable. Midwife and scholar Betty Anne Daviss argues that if the success of the social movement is defined as the protection of home birth and informed choice for women, then professional midwifery can be said to have succeeded. However, she fears that the spirit of the original movement has been eroded as professional midwives cease to challenge aspects of the mainstream system. She maintains a distinction between the success of professional midwifery and the larger alternative birth movement, which has more diverse goals and participants than professional midwifery (2001, 81–82).

What is clear is that midwifery meant different things to different people involved. Midwives wanted to pursue regulation and public funding for various reasons. Many were tired of being marginal and poorly remunerated for their work, others were tired of being seen as "crazy radicals," and many were committed to the greater access to midwifery care that legitimacy and public funding would provide. The decision to seek incorporation was contested, and divisions within the OAM remained as the process gained momentum. The OAM and the ONMA collaborated on a single submission to the HPLR as the Midwifery Coalition, and eventually these two groups merged to form the Association of Ontario Midwives (AOM). The AOM continues to be the professional body representing midwives and the practice of midwifery in Ontario. According to Van Wagner, "the strategy of the midwifery movement [was] to create a highly visible practice outside of the health care system while pressuring for legislation, autonomy, government funding, and access for all women" (1988: 115).

Once the decision to pursue incorporation into the health care system had been made, the Midwifery Task Force of Ontario (MTF-O) was formed in 1983 as a separate organization to represent consumers and other midwifery supporters. It became "an organized voice" of families calling for changes to maternity care, and members were involved in fundraising and public education about midwifery. The official mandate of the MTF-O was to lobby for the recognition and incorporation of midwifery. This organization was instrumental in midwifery gaining legal and professional status.[11] The bureaucratic reorganization of midwifery at this time—specifically, the amalgamation of nurse- and non-nurse midwives and the separation of midwifery and consumer organizations—was a critical strategy toward the goal of incorporation (Bourgeault 2006, 83–84).

Why now in Ontario? Robin, a long practicing, politically active midwife sums it up this way:

A relatively good number of very hard-working, very sane midwives and very hard-working and sane consumers. I honestly think it's that simple on some level. I also think that the fact that it had very clear political unification under one agenda is absolutely critical. That's why in some of the States (even though midwifery has been around with the same history as here) it has just gone down the tubes. People there couldn't agree on standards, all those kind of things. Having to politically make midwifery an option for people and making us define it in a way that the public could understand with clear standards is what made midwifery [in Ontario] happen . . . I would say—and of course you know I'm biased—the fact is, that there has been a reasonable number of people who are fairly pragmatic.

While the union of nurse-midwives and non–nurse-midwives under the AOM was politically strategic, it was not without conflict and dissent and some ironies of its own. Ingrid, for example, was trained as a nurse-midwife outside of Canada in a system that she readily admits was a "very medical model." Shortly after she arrived in Canada in the early 1980s and discovered that there was no professional midwifery, she started a home birth practice. While she was, in her words, "sympathetic to the cause" of professionalization of midwifery in Ontario she was not a member of the AOM during this time because, in her experience,

it was beginning to place a lot of restrictions on midwifery. It was like, VBACs couldn't be done at home and if you belonged to the AOM you couldn't do them. And I didn't agree with that. So I used to do VBACs at home if I wanted to. I didn't buy that thing of being dictated to.[12]

Though she was determined and confident to practice midwifery outside AOM standards, Ingrid does not see herself as radical. On the contrary, she felt that the AOM at the time was too radical for her: "You had to be all for the cause . . . like a very strong feminist movement, which was great, but you had to abide by the rules and fit into their concept of what midwifery was. And all I wanted to do was be a midwife and deliver babies." Ingrid's experience highlights some of the curious tensions and competing visions within midwifery at the time. Paradoxically, Ingrid found herself not radical enough to belong to the AOM, an organization that was beginning to place restrictions on midwifery as a radical practice.

In October 1992, a pre-registration program designed to bring into the system midwives already practicing in the community was set in place at the Michener Institute of Applied Health Sciences in Toronto. An international faculty was recruited from Denmark, the Netherlands, Britain, and New Zealand to assess the candidates, and 71 of 120 applicants were admitted to the program. In October 1993, sixty-three of these graduated and became the first Registered Midwives in the province and, indeed, the country. The Michener Pre-registration Program generated a great deal of controversy and criticism among midwives and their consumers and supporters for a number of reasons. First, nine of the sixty-three experienced community midwives received "incomplete" assessments, with no mechanisms in place to complete them. After a period of intense lobbying by these midwives and consumer supporters in their home communities, the Michener Program was extended to permit these midwives to complete it as well. Second, a group called the Committee for More Midwives (CMM) sprang up to fight against what they perceived to be an unacceptable situation for midwives with experience but who were not considered experienced enough to be admitted to the pre-registration program.[13]

The successful process by which midwifery was transformed from a grassroots social movement into a regulated profession involved certain restrictions on practice and the suppression of differences between midwives—part of the shadow story of professionalization I wrote about in Chapter 1. Ingrid is by no means alone. Other midwives also felt silenced or marginalized during the time leading up to incorporation, and yet most acknowledge that it was necessary to present a unified front to the HPLR, and few feel that it could have happened any other way. Ingrid lauds the hard work and determination of what she describes as "the strongest group of women you've ever seen" in achieving for everyone what she considers to be the best midwifery system in the world.

The New Midwifery and Health System Integration

Midwifery was declared a legal profession in Ontario on January 1, 1994, and the process of incorporating this new profession into the health care system intensified. Ontario midwifery is defined in accordance with the international definition of a midwife:[14]

> The practice of midwifery is the assessment and monitoring of women during pregnancy, labour and the post-partum period and of their newborn babies, the provision of care during normal pregnancy, labour and the post-partum period and the conducting of spontaneous normal vaginal deliveries. (Midwifery Act 1991)

Midwifery is now accessible to all women in Ontario who are experiencing normal, uncomplicated pregnancy and birth. The total number of midwives in Ontario has grown from fifty in the mid-1990s to more than 300 today. Midwives attend approximately 8 percent of all births in the province, and the province plans to expand the availability of midwifery services as the demand continues to grow. All midwives must register with the College of Midwives of Ontario (CMO), the governing body whose mandate it is to administer the Midwifery Act in the public interest. The Association of Ontario Midwives represents the professional interests of Registered Midwives (RMs). Meanwhile, the MTF-O lives on as the Ontario Midwifery Consumers Network (OMCN) with a new mandate to preserve and promote the Ontario model of midwifery care. OMCN members are now involved in public education about midwifery and sit as representatives on local and provincial committees that govern the practice of midwifery.

Most midwives work in practice groups made up of between two and eight practitioners. A small number of solo midwives work in rural areas, with a provision for the use of second attendants who are not registered midwives but may in some cases be nurses. Many midwives combine their clinical work with work in the College of Midwives and the Association of Ontario Midwives, and faculty positions in the Midwifery Education Program (MEP). When compared with other jurisdictions in Canada, the United States, and abroad, midwifery in Ontario is structurally unique in several ways. First, it is a direct-entry profession (one need not become a nurse first). Second, it is fully funded by the provincial health care system, meaning that women can access midwifery services at no direct cost to themselves.[15] Third, midwives are primary care providers who follow their own clients from pregnancy through labor and delivery and up to six weeks post-partum rather than work on shifts in hospitals or as subordinates to physicians. This also means that midwives have hospital admitting and discharging privileges. Fourth, midwifery in Ontario allows choice of birth place, including home birth. In the sections below I address each of these aspects of midwifery in turn.

Midwifery Education

Despite recommendations from the nursing and medical professions that prior nursing training be a prerequisite for midwifery education, the AOM successfully argued for a direct-entry model. Thus, entrance to the Ontario Midwifery Education Program does not require a prior degree in nursing or health sciences. A university rather than college setting for midwifery education was also seen as critical be-cause, as the Midwifery Task Force reasoned, hospitals would be un-likely to grant admitting and discharging privileges to anyone with less than a Bachelor's of Science and thus midwives' educational credentials would have a major bearing on their legitimacy as prac-titioners and their ability to offer choice of birth place (Bourgeault 2006: 162).

The four-year BSc Midwifery Education Program (MEP) oper-ates at three university sites in Ontario.[16] It is comprised of a rigorous academic component and a series of clinical placements with practic-ing midwives and physicians in order to combine standardized aca-demic qualifications with an apprenticeship approach to learning. The faculty are largely practicing midwives, most of whom have advanced degrees. Midwifery education and training further depends on the participation of practicing midwives and their clients. Midwives across the province act as preceptors to midwifery students, and because the profession is still relatively small, most have a fairly constant rotation of students with them. Likewise, most women in midwifery care in Ontario are encouraged to accommodate a student midwife. The first class of midwives graduated from the MEP in September 1996, and the program continues to draw a large number of applications for relatively few spots each year. Between September 1993 (its inception) and the fall of 2002, 153 students had completed the program (Kaufman and Soderstrom 2004). The total number of graduates each year from the three campuses has increased from eighteen in 1996 to over forty in 2004, and the goal for the coming years is to graduate at least sixty new midwives per year. Standardized education is literally changing the face of midwifery in Ontario. It is interesting to note that more than two-thirds of the midwives currently registered in the province have graduated within the last ten years.

Access to the profession is also possible through the International Midwifery Pre-registration Program (IMPP), which assesses the qualification of midwives trained in other jurisdictions in Canada and abroad, and stipulates a process for meeting the criteria for registration in Ontario.[17] Ontario midwives are promoting their direct-entry BSc education model, which will streamline reciprocity in terms of registering midwives trained in other provinces. The Midwifery Act in Ontario also includes an exemption for Aboriginal midwives. As a consequence, Aboriginal midwives may be accredited by internal criteria and are able to serve other Aboriginal women in their communities.[18] The creation of these multiple routes to midwifery education and registration are significant in creating access to the profession. Given the cultural and linguistic diversity of the province, the need to diversify the profession has been evident since the beginning.[19] In addition, steps have been taken since legislation to actively recruit women of color into the profession through the Midwifery Education Program. With these steps, ethnic and linguistic diversity within the profession is increasing.

Midwifery Funding

Midwifery services are accessible through the Ontario Health Insurance Program (OHIP), the mechanism by which all Ontarions access health care at no direct cost to themselves. Women simply present their OHIP card to their choice of primary maternity care provider at their first appointment: midwife, family physician, or OB/GYN. Midwives do not bill on a fee-for-service basis as do physicians; rather, they are paid a salary for fulfilling a requisite number of courses of care per year. A full-time midwife attends forty births per year as the primary midwife and forty births per year as the "second" midwife. (There are two midwives at every birth; the primary midwife arrives first and attends throughout the labor and delivery, while the second arrives when the birth is imminent). Midwifery has been shown to be cost-effective maternity care, compared to obstetrician care or family physician care. First, normal births are not handled by specialists whose services cost the province more. Second, home births do not require the use of hospital beds and services, such as meals and housekeeping. Third, planned hospital-birth clients typically leave the hospital sooner because midwives provide at-home postpartum care. And fourth, midwifery is associated with less technology and medication use during labor as well as lower rates of interventions both in hospital and at home (Johnson and Daviss 2005).

Ideally, public funding makes midwifery care accessible to diverse cultural, linguistic, and religious communities. Practices across the province typically advertise the range of languages spoken. Further, midwifery practices are developing ways to outreach and adapt their work to the particular needs of various groups in their communities: teenage mothers, incarcerated mothers, non-status immigrants, and low-income families. Some of these outreach activities are funded by other Ministry of Health programs, such as funds for language translation and services to non-status immigrants with no health care coverage.

Health System Integration

The integration of midwifery into the Ontario heath care system might be described diplomatically as "a learning process" involving "growing pains." The opposition to midwifery prior to legislation did not dissolve overnight. Especially in the early years, many physicians and nurses strenuously objected to the professional autonomy of midwives and their rates of remuneration, and questioned their training and skills. The process for obtaining hospital privileges was not adapted well for midwives in all places. Physicians quite rightly complained that a payment system for their consulting work with midwifery clients was not in place when midwives were initially brought on. Some physicians directed their anger toward midwives rather than their college or the province, who failed to address the problem in a timely manner; a few physicians went so far as to refuse to consult with midwives at all, effectively denying local specialist care to midwifery clients.

It is worth noting that midwives became the only health professionals in the last one hundred years to gain hospital admitting and discharging privileges—something previously held exclusively by physicians and dental surgeons. (Privileges are essential to midwifery autonomy and their ability to offer choice of birth place.) The presence of midwifery as a new profession in the hospital was particularly challenging for all parties; it meant changes to provincial legislation like the Hospitals Act, and it meant changes to individual hospitals' internal protocols and departments. Physicians, nurses, and hospitals were not always welcoming to midwives and were sometimes openly hostile. This chilly reception was partly due to the changes they felt were pressed upon them, but it also has a history. Prior to legislation, many nurses and physicians were not only opposed to midwifery as an idea but also may have been witness to what they saw as "midwifery disasters" and "botched home births," while failing to see these transfers to hospital as appropriate (Davis-Floyd 2003) and while having little knowledge of midwife-attended home births that went perfectly well. Many midwives who practiced prior to integration, for their part, had come from a position of being critical of hospitals and the standard approaches to childbirth taken by the nurses and doctors who worked there. Many were not comfortable in hospitals and did not easily take to the routines and bureaucratic requirements. Nursing staff, for their part, were concerned about the implications of this new profession for their job security and their turf in the hospital. They were frustrated in everyday ways, too, when midwives could not remember routines or paperwork, or where to find supplies. Overall, midwifery integration varied across the province. While in some Ontario hospitals, nurses and physicians have welcomed midwives and the new approach to maternity care that they bring, in other hospitals physicians and midwives appear locked in bitter battles that are troubling to them as professionals and persons and to the public as well.[20]

The Midwifery Model of Care

The Ontario midwifery model of care is designed to be continuous and personalized, to involve the wishes and shared responsibility of the birthing woman, and to strive to support a woman to "give birth safely with power and with dignity" (CMO 1994, 1). This intention is manifested in a clinical model that emphasizes the consumer-oriented principles of continuity of care, choice of birth place, and informed choice. Midwives, while autonomous primary care providers, work within a network of other health professionals and services. They requisition blood work and ultrasounds from medical labs. They consult with family physicians, obstetricians, neonatologists, and pediatricians when medical conditions or circumstances arise for their mothers or newborns that fall outside the midwifery scope of practice. For example, if a client develops high blood pressure during pregnancy, she must consult with an obstetrician and may require a transfer of care; if the condition is resolved, the care may be transferred back to the midwife. The presence of twins, however, causes an automatic irreversible transfer of care to an obstetrician. Consults and transfers can occur during labor, delivery, or the postpartum period. A request for the pharmaceutical augmentation of labor or an epidural for pain relief, for example, typically requires a transfer of care, though some midwives and physicians would like to see this changed.

Despite variations in backgrounds, training, and philosophical orientations among Ontario community midwives, most reiterate the importance of the three principles of informed choice, continuity of care, and choice of birth place. The relative importance they place on these three pillars of midwifery care, however, varies. A rural midwife, Katherine, remarks:

> The very most important thing is the choice of birth place. Absolutely. The only other country that says you have choice of birth place is, in my mind, Holland. We offer it here, and it's not just lip service to a choice. I think that is completely and totally unique. I think the way we work in small on-call practice groups to offer continuity is another huge hallmark of midwifery in Ontario. And if you have ever seen the AOM cup with the three leaves of the trillium—that [image represents] informed choice, choice of birth place, and continuity of care. They are the things that are totally different than the way things are in other jurisdictions—even as close as the United States. We have a very strong model that's actually been regulated. Professions get regulated, but we've managed to say that in order to have midwifery and have it do what you want it to do for your health care system—reduce costs, increase better outcomes—then what you have to do is let it have a strong core, or a strong model. So they have actually governed that by having two primary care providers at every birth, by saying you must give the woman the choice, by ensuring that choice availability is there. That's what's really different [about midwifery in Ontario].

Another midwife, Laura, concurs by reflecting on why she became a midwife in the first place, and why midwifery developed as a social and political movement. Laura was self-trained and practiced for many years outside the system in Canada and prior to that in the United States. She is now in her early fifties and works in a large urban center.

Well, the reason that we all started doing this was because of home birth. There were no caregivers for home birth. And most of us also were women in that time who had home births ourselves. I really felt that I was stepping out on a limb, doing something that was not legal because I felt very strongly about preserving that. So therefore, logically, if I had been told that I could only work in the hospital now I probably would have kept doing home births rather than become a legal midwife.

As midwifery legislation is introduced across the country, Ontario midwives are hoping that all provinces will implement a model of midwifery that allows home birth. Even as the debate continues to unfold about midwifery and home birth, the first clinical studies including Canadian data have been published (Janssen et al 2002: Johnson and Daviss 2005). The positive results in terms of the safety of home birth, client satisfaction, and cost savings to the health care system may increase the likelihood of home birth being part of midwifery in others provinces as well.[21]

Informed Choice

Other midwives stress that informed choice is the most unique and important aspect of the Ontario midwifery model of care. The principle of informed choice in midwifery is based on the notion that women can and should understand the rationale behind different courses of action in their maternity care and thus be in a position to share the responsibility of making important decisions about their own care. Informed choice in midwifery is similar to informed consent in medical-legal and ethical terms; it is designed to protect patient autonomy and one's right to exercise control over one's own body. It obliges clinicians to fully inform patients of all risks, benefits, and alternatives to procedures. Moreover, it prohibits clinicians from imposing treatment on competent individuals even if such treatment is deemed life saving (Faulder 1985 in Kaufert and O'Neil 1989, 42).

Yet the principle of informed choice in the midwifery model of care differs from informed consent in at least two significant ways.

First, informed choice is an inherently politicized notion, given the centrality of choice as an organizing concept and goal of the broader women's health movement, of which midwifery is a part. Midwives often told me that their initial interest in becoming midwives was to offer women choices in childbirth. The depth of their commitment to this political agenda sustained many of them through the years of legal, political, financial, and personal instability that characterized midwifery in the 1980s and early 1990s.

Second, whereas the ideal of informed consent is circumscribed by the way that medicine is typically practiced, informed choice is facilitated by other key aspects of midwifery philosophy and clinical practice. Specifically, informed choice in midwifery care is under-pinned by a philosophy that challenges the hierarchical authority of biomedicine and what is perceived as an over reliance on technology. Midwives strive instead for a more egalitarian client relationship in which low-tech ways of knowing and doing are explored and valued. Continuity of care (having the same primary care givers through-out) and long appointments encourage trust to develop between the midwife and client and allow time for the client's own knowledge to come out.

Midwives have the time to share and discuss with their clients the latest scientific evidence. They also tend to consider nonscientific in-formation—a woman's own knowledge, feelings, and past experiences about her body and previous pregnancies, as well as her lifestyle and moral and religious beliefs. By way of a quick example, one woman in my study was extremely averse to giving birth in the same hospital where she had witnessed two family members die in recent months. Her midwife considered this important information that could affect her birthing process, and together they planned a home birth. An-other woman in my study was from a medical family—her father and father-in-law were doctors, while she herself was a teacher—and for her, it was the opportunity to study and discuss statistics on the safety of home versus hospital birth that enabled her to make what she felt was a truly informed decision with regard to her choice of birth place. Midwives try not to tell women what to do as long as the situation falls within their scope of practice and is not a life threatening emergency. (Though there is some debate over how far informed choice should go). They encourage clients to fully share the responsibilities of making choices about their care, even if they are reluctant to do so. As one midwife told me, "If a woman is saying to me 'Oh, I don't know. You tell me what to do' I just keep putting it back to her." Midwives in my study did note, however, that some clients are still reluctant to reproduce the ideal egalitarian midwife-client relationship that prevailed before legislation.

Thus the principle of informed choice cannot be separated from the broader political pursuit of women's choices in childbirth. Nor does it operate independently of other midwifery fundamentals. Midwife Laura insists firmly and simply that "having time with women" is what promotes and safeguards truly informed choice. In the words of another midwife-activist, "Midwives need autonomy to give women autonomy" (Van Wagner in Bourgeault 2006, 147). Yet sociologist Ivy Bourgeault, who has conducted an in-depth study of the process of professionalization (2006), argues that the new system of midwifery as a self-regulating profession rather than as a consumer-driven and regulated one does curtail consumer input to some degree. Certainly, midwifery in Ontario has been clinically limited by regulation. For example, midwives must decline to care for women carrying twins or delivering a baby in a breech presentation, as these situations fall outside their scope of practice. Yet, at the same time, midwifery has been expanded by regulation to include such things as ordering prenatal diagnostic tests and inserting IVs in hospitals and at home to administer fluids and prophylactic antibiotics during labor. While a few birthing women actively resist the limitations placed on their choices by midwifery regulation, more commonly midwives voice discomfort over providing certain services that were not formerly part of midwifery.[22]

The third pillar of the Ontario midwifery model of care is continuity of care, though fewer midwives cite it as most important. Continuity of care means that the same midwife sees a woman through her entire pregnancy, birth, and postpartum period, including for newborn care. To accomplish this, midwives have extended on-call hours—often weeks at a time. Continuity of care is perhaps the most difficult aspect of the midwifery model to carry out, and midwives now admit to a degree of idealism in pressing this as a central part of the model. While continuity of care is one of the most appealing aspects of midwifery care from the perspective of birthing women, it creates a "caring dilemma" for midwives (Benoit 1998). How can they balance their personal lives with the tremendous amount of time and caring they give their clients?

When midwives worked outside of the system, they did not have the volume of births they do now nor the added responsibilities of sitting on hospital committees, training students, or many other professional duties. Some midwifery practice groups have now instituted variations on continuity of care—such as working in small, shared-care teams of three or four midwives for each client, so that each client can be sure to have two midwives that she knows at her birth, and so that midwives can have more time off-call. The model of midwifery care in Ontario is not set in stone. Midwifery still has many challenges from within and without to maintain its current scope of practice and funding situation within the system. Laura's view of the current state of midwifery in Ontario reveals a tension between celebration and caution—an awareness that the favorable position of midwifery in the health care system is not guaranteed.

> Compared to what I know about other places, we do have certain things that are written in and protected but are manipulatable in some ways. One thing right now that I think is especially unique is that we have so much time with women. The government at this point has funded us this way and at some point they are going to get wind of this and say "Those midwives don't need 45 minutes with clients. There's no proof!" And so for us, are we going to have to be able to show that we have a need for such long visits? And so for me the luxury that still remains is the time we have with women. But you know that's not one of the official philosophies of midwifery care. [The official philosophy] is continuity of care and normal birth and home birth and women's choice is protected . . . If the time we have with women is not protected, then women's choice will not be protected.

In other words, the simple practice of spending time with women is critical to ensuring informed choice and choice of birth place—the two more overtly political aspects of the midwifery model of care, and the two most often mentioned by midwives as the most important aspects of midwifery in Ontario.

New Tales, New Tasks

The story of midwifery in Ontario is a remarkable one. Having overcome a history of denigration, trenchant opposition from physicians, and threats of usurpation from the nursing profession, the grassroots social movement of midwifery—peopled predominantly by women, no less—becomes a fully incorporated health profession, winning political sanction, public funding, and a growing acceptance by the public. The face of maternity care in Canada is changed irrevocably. But if it can be considered a renaissance, it is an elaborate one, still marked by the shadow stories of professionalization and the persistent growing pains of the first decade of incorporation. In this chapter I have offered historical and sociological context for the more anthropological description and analysis to come. I will return to some of the material presented here in the next chapter, where, for example, I explore the uses to which these historical interpretations and sociological definitions have been put by midwives and birthing women in an effort to illuminate midwifery identity. Later, in Chapters 4 and 5, I go on to show how these historical and sociological definitions affect the embodied experiences of midwifery clients as well.

CHAPTER THREE

What is Midwifery?

What is found at the historical beginning of things is not the inviolable identity of their origin; it is the dissension of other things (Foucault 1984, 79).

AMONG THE MOST POPULAR ideas about the new midwifery in Canada is that it is the resurrection of an ancient, universal tradition of women helping women in childbirth—a kind of maternal nurture, a natural extension of domestic healing roles. Other descriptions have focused more on midwifery as a social change movement devoted to the demedicalization of childbirth and the re-empowerment of women through childbirth. Both definitions posit midwifery as a radical alternative to "technocratic birth" (Davis-Floyd 1997). The first describes midwifery in terms of tradition and universality while the second sees it in terms of overt resistance—two prime anthropological themes.

My concern in this chapter is to explore midwifery identity in Ontario through the retelling and analysis of midwifery narratives—stories of becoming and being a midwife, and stories of seeking out and experiencing midwifery care. In these stories, midwifery emerges as a complex cultural system that is certainly influenced by discourses of history, universality, and resistance but is ultimately invented in the present and shaped by its participants out of present-day ideological and clinical concerns. The present location of midwifery within the formal health care system, for example, has altered its content and status as a tradition or as a social movement in significant ways. Further, following legislation and incorporation, midwifery has increasingly been described simply as the work of midwives: the set of clinical knowledge and practices having to do with pregnancy and childbirth, falling within a specified scope of practice and carried out within a defined professional setting. Indeed, it was a critically important time to foreground this clinical or professional identity over what might be described as other ideological or analytical identities—meanings of midwifery that speak to its social and political intentions.

When I refer to the ideological or analytical identity of midwifery I am pointing to the inseparability of ethnographic data and anthropological analysis. As Kirin Narayan points out, "narratives are not transparent representations of what actually happened, but are told for particular purposes, from particular points of view: they are thus incipiently analytical, enacting theory (1997, 36). On this note I begin this chapter with a section called Essential Reading which explores the relationship between midwifery identity and childbirth literature—both popular and scholarly. It may seem like a digression or even part of a literature review, rather than a piece of the ethnographic setting, but reading has been central to midwifery's ideological and practical development, thus informing the "particular view" from which the midwifery narratives are experienced and told.

The rest of the chapter pursues a descriptive and analytical strategy in which I explore a series of questions. To what extent does contemporary Canadian midwifery resemble its historical and cross-cultural counterparts? Should midwifery be read as the renaissance of an ancient tradition? An extension of maternal nurture? Or should midwifery be read primarily in terms of resistance to biomedicine and technocratic birth? Beyond these familiar questions, I also critically explore whether and how midwifery might be understood as a hybrid of science and medicine on the one hand and of nature and feminism on the other.

Essential Reading

Most midwives and their clients in Ontario read books for inspiration and information. Michel Odent's *Childbirth without Fear,* Ina Mae Gaskin's *Spiritual Midwifery,* Raven Lang's *Birth Book,* Sheila Kitzinger's *Home Birth,* and Suzanne Arms's *Immaculate Deception* were part of the canon of Canadian community midwifery as it reemerged in the minds and meeting spaces across the country where aspiring midwives came together in study groups.[1] Most midwives cite reading as essential to their development as practitioners and activists. Sonja, for example, started her midwifery practice from scratch in a rural area in Ontario in the early 1980s. She had a home birth for her first baby and was a breastfeeding advocate and counselor in her community, but she had no real contact with the larger midwifery community that was beginning to organize for change around that time. What she knew about midwifery came from her own experience and from books.

> What I knew about midwifery was mainly what I had read—
> books like Suzanne Arms and Sheila Kitzinger, who is definitely
> a very good spokesperson. I knew the British model and had
> this very comforting vision of the British midwife who knows
> everything, does everything [because it] is a long-standing
> tradition in Britain. It was an interesting contrast to what I
> knew about American midwifery from reading books like
> *Spiritual Midwifery* by Ina Mae Gaskin—sort of the rediscovery
> of midwifery from the ground up. So what I have is a real
> hodgepodge of approaches to midwifery. And I think what we
> are trying to do [here in Ontario] is some kind of blending of
> well-grounded clinical stuff with the flexible, woman-centered
> approach of the sort of hippie-centered tradition of midwives
> in North America. They really grasped on to the laid-back,
> everything is normal, everything is natural approach . . . I think
> that is probably the way a lot of us started.

Sonja's vision for midwifery—a very Canadian blend of British/
European sensibility and American individualism—was remarkably

widespread. Years later, many of these same books are still read by midwives and their clients in Ontario. Every midwifery clinic in the province boasts an impressive lending library of books and magazines about midwifery and birth. Indeed, self-education through reading is one of the central prescriptions of midwifery care, and clients typically mentioned books as one of their key sources of information, inspiration, and politicization about pregnancy and birth. Three-time midwifery client, Anna Lisa, spontaneously drew in her reading to respond to my question about why she had chosen to give birth at home:

> I don't know. I was trying to be a rebel or something. It *did* make sense to me that you should have your first in the hospital, and then I read Sheila Kitzinger's *Birth at Home,* and that really sold me. It just seemed so simple; just that, like, everybody's doing it all over the world. Its been going on for thousands of years.

Essential reading in midwifery (in addition to studying standard medical manuals) was of two kinds: popular alternative childbirth literature, which tended to be feminist oriented, and physician-authored alternative birth manuals. Both drew on nostalgic notions of natural birth experienced by traditional non-Western women, inspired in part by works in the anthropology of midwifery and childbirth. Indeed, I suggest that there has been a close, productive—even formative—relationship between anthropological scholarship and midwifery and alternative childbirth books. As childbirth alternatives—including independent forms of midwifery—were taking shape amid the sweeping social changes underway in Europe and North America in the 1970s, anthropologists were studying and writing about midwifery and childbirth elsewhere. In the late 1970s and early 1980s came a wave of ethnographic studies by professional anthropologists who took as their focus non-Western birthing systems and addressed the wide range of beliefs and practices surrounding conception, pregnancy, and birth in Western and non-Western settings (Cosminsky 1976, 1977; Jordan 1993 [1978], 1987; Kay 1982; Laderman 1983; McClain 1975, 1981, 1982; MacCormack 1982; Sargent 1989). This body of work established reproduction as a socially, culturally, and politically significant phenomenon.

In this literature, the traditional or indigenous midwife often appears as an ancestral figure, the bearer of the social and cultural tradition of midwifery, as well as a repository of clinical knowledge about the natural facts of pregnancy and birth. Birthing women in other times and places appear as knowledgeable, self-sufficient, physically strong, and close to nature. (Scholars too have been drawn into the romance of the authentic, often keenly aware of the power of such symbols to establish particular claims.) The anthropological image of traditional or indigenous midwifery as a universal (but culturally specific) woman-centered tradition, which relies on simple or "appropriate" technology to aid the "natural" process of birth, took on iconic status in the alternative childbirth literature of this time.[2] Consider the opening pages of sociologist Suzanne Arms's alternative childbirth classic *Immaculate Deception* (1975).

> Imagine your distant ancestor, living in a small village on the edge of a forest. She is a member of a small group of hunters and food gatherers. The time is late summer, when days are warm but nights are chilly. This young woman is ready to give birth . . . The midwife comes, a woman in middle life, her black hair beginning to gray. Carrying her birth tools in a small pouch over her arm, she greets the young woman with an appraising look . . . (1–3)

In building this nostalgic image, Arms uses the work of anthropologist Margaret Mead (1972, 8–9) to establish her claims about what birth was like for "primitive women." Arms's thesis is that Christianity and "civilization" have built a modern deception about childbirth—that it is inherently dangerous, defiling, and horribly painful. Consequently, North American women approach childbirth with a tremendous fear of pain, loss of control, and loss of dignity. The image of a natural birth attended by a traditional midwife symbolically condenses her important message that we in the West have strayed from a state of nature but that a return is possible and necessary. The main body of her book describes such a return already underway in the home birth movement in North America and serves as a call to arms for women to get involved.

Sheila Kitzinger is an anthropologist, childbirth educator, advisor to the national Childbirth Trust in Great Britain, and one of the most influential childbirth educators in the English-speaking world. She also employs anthropological data about diverse birthing practices in a series of popular books to argue that we in the West have lost our awareness of birth as an important life event and that we have become culturally impoverished because of it.[3] Kitzinger argues that with home birth, women and families can regain the joy and a sense of responsibility for their bodies, their pregnancies, and their births (1980). Though she believes that home birth may not be for everyone, the knowledge of the existence of alternatives to medicalized births in hospitals, she argues, is essential to improving the dominant system for all women (1980). In *The Midwife Challenge* (1988), Kitzinger evokes images of ancient midwives, quoting from anthropological texts as well as such sources as the Tao Te Ching and ancient Egyptian papyri to establish the universal antiquity of midwifery. She calls on midwives to become aware of the worldwide challenge for them to reconnect to the ancient art of midwifery while simultaneously evolving a new one (1988).

Elisabeth Barrington, author of *Midwifery is Catching* (1985), the first popular book about the new midwifery in Canada—and a book read widely by midwives and clients alike—is clearly aware of this literature when she writes:

> Recently, people have been discovering that in other places, and under different care systems, some parents have it better. The consumer movement has made information about alternatives readily available, and the midwifery movement provides a model for comparison. (20)

Barrington illustrates her point in a discussion about the custom of leaving women to labor almost entirely alone—a practice unique to North American obstetrics, she notes. "Social anthropologists," she remarks, "point out that even among primitive tribes, our custom would be pronounced barbaric. Such is the lonely heart of Canadian childbirth culture" (1985, 21).

Indeed, anthropologists at the same time were documenting a diversity of birthing systems and comparing them favorably to the Western way. Anthropologist Brigitte Jordan's classic *Birth in Four Cultures,* for example, first published in 1978, has been received by a scholarly and a popular audience. Jordan compares and contrasts specific elements of birthing systems in the United States, Holland, Sweden, and Mexico, and explicitly intended her work to serve as a critique of the "American way of birth." For example, she observed how Mayan *parteras* provide emotional support during labor and suggests that this part of maternity care has been vastly undervalued in the West (1993, 67). Jordan wrote of the "need to go outside American obstetrics, both to un-medicalized birthing systems within American culture and to the indigenous systems of the Third and Fourth Worlds for generating alternatives to its rigidity and standardization—an enterprise with increasing importance as the American model gains ascendance in the developing world" (1993, 145).

Of birthing women themselves, social scientists observed that many non-Western women enjoyed a high degree of autonomy and control over their births. The hallmark of comparative anthropological studies of birth in the 1980s is captured in Laderman's conclusion that "the essential difference between childbirth in America and childbirth in Merchang is clear. American women are delivered by obstetricians; Merchang women give birth" (1983, 173). Anthropological studies of reproduction in biomedical systems of the West have supported this assertion from the other side (Davis-Floyd 1992, 1994; Davis-Floyd and Davis 1997; Martin 1987; Fraser 1995; Michaelson 1988; Romalis 1982). Robbie Davis-Floyd's well-known ethnography *Birth as an American Rite of Passage* (1992) is representative. She argues that childbirth as a rite of passage consists of highly ritualized practices that divest women of any power they might feel and redirect it into the hands of hospital staff (1988, 157). Women are made to think of their bodies as weak, disabled, unclean, defective machines and are led to believe that their only hope for themselves and their babies is to relinquish all control to the institution. Ultimately, this rite of passage initiates women into the core values of American culture: technology, progress, standardization.[4] In a more recent work Davis-Floyd uses the term "technocratic birth" to describe the constellation of ideas, institutional and clinical practices, and effects that characterize modern obstetrical medicine and, significantly, what is viewed to be its generally negative effect on women as individuals and as a group (1994). Importantly, though with less detail, Davis-Floyd also describes how women sometimes resist or appropriate their initiation. Overall, these scholarly anthropological works reveal a political agenda of childbirth reform in North America, its alternative vision—and sometimes its technology—fueled by studies of birthing systems in other times and places.[5] Brigitte Jordan makes a point of comparing American birth to traditional low-tech midwifery among the Maya of the Yucatan peninsula as well as to birth in the high-tech hospitals of Sweden.

Another genre of essential reading in the re-emergence of midwifery was the physician-authored natural childbirth manual epitomized by Grantly Dick-Read's *Childbirth without Fear* (1959). According to Dick-Read, "In natural childbirth the body performs its task unencumbered by fearful expectation" (quoted in Livingstone 1993, 347–348). "Cultural birth," in contrast, involves great fear and expectation of childbirth pain, which alters the natural physiological process. Dick-Read supposed that cultural birth would give way to natural birth if women were properly educated and supported in childbirth. French obstetrician Michel Odent's particular version of "natural childbirth" has been equally influential. Based on observations in his own birthing clinic in Pithiviers, France, and his study of birth "in other cultures," Odent posits a universal basis to birth. He believes that, given the right environment, women can transcend their cultural upbringing and connect with their natural birthing instincts. But, he observes, women must be educated and supported in doing so (1984). The themes of education, relaxation, and support for birthing women as the means to achieve natural childbirth continue to underpin social and psychological studies of labor and parturition, as well as most methods of prepared childbirth (Livingstone 1993, 348).[6]

Thus have "other mothers" (Nestel 1995) and other midwiferies become essential reading—imaginary spaces and persons consumed by contemporary midwifery as objects of desire—ancestral figures, custodians of special knowledge about pregnancy and birth that can be reincorporated into contemporary birth culture. Much more has and could be said on this topic regarding both negative and potentially positive evaluations of such cultural appropriation, but my purpose here is to show how such perspectives assume an essential association between women and nature, to examine how that association has been employed to unify women against universal patriarchy, and to posit a basis for women's empowerment.[7]

Midwifery and Maternal Nurture

> Fieldnote, Sept. 12, 1996: A conversation in the waiting room. Ingrid is boasting to a client on her way out that the midwives at this practice have many children amongst them: Laura has two, Gwen has five, Sarah has four, Marguerite is pregnant with her third, and she herself has five. "Having children is like a form of professional development for midwives," she says. It reminds me of what Bridget (another midwife in another practice) told me last week: "I know that this is politically incorrect, but I believe that midwives should be mothers."

Ought midwifery be construed as the re-emergence of an ancient tradition of women helping women in childbirth? Is midwifery in Ontario based primarily on maternal nurture and as an extension of domestic healing roles? The fact that in the mid-1990s most midwives in Ontario *were* mothers might lend weight to such an argument. The classic profile of a midwife established in the anthropological and historical literature is that of an older woman who comes to know about childbirth through a combination of personal experience and empirical observation, and then turns to assist other women in her community. As Ehrenreich and English have written, "The art of healing has always been linked to the tasks and spirit of motherhood: wisdom, nurturance, tenderness, skill" (1978, 34). Emphasizing a link between motherhood and healing is one way that women have been recognized and affirmed as healers in anthropological and historical studies when prior work tended to exclude their mention (McClain 1989).[8] But to what extent does contemporary midwifery in Ontario resemble its historical and cross-cultural counterparts? Asking this question is an analytical strategy, rather than an attempt to establish this interpretation.

Midwives in Ontario differ widely from the classic midwife profile in the anthropological literature: they range in age from mid-twenties, to mid-seventies (most are in their thirties, forties, and fifties); they range in marital status and sexual orientation; they range in parental responsibilities from having no children at all, to being single mothers of young children, parents of grown children, and grandparents. They are not all in heterosexual relationships nor traditional nuclear families. There was one male midwife in Ontario who has since left the province; he worked with his female partner before legislation and graduated from the Michener Program with the first batch of professional midwives in 1993. The MEP has received a number of applications from men wanting to become midwives; though none have been admitted as yet, it may be just a matter of time. Studies of independent midwifery in the United States note a similar demographic profile (Sullivan and Weitz 1988).

Maternal nurture *is* part of the story for many midwives, and the sense that the principles, values, and work of mothering is crucial to the health of women, children, and families does form part of the expectations of midwifery for the women they attend. Reflecting on why they had chosen midwifery, or why they preferred it to physician care, many of the women in my study told me about their mothers' experiences of childbirth. Because most of the women I interviewed were in their twenties and thirties, their mothers—having given birth in the late 1950s, 1960s and early 1970s—are of a generation that had fewer choices in childbirth.[9] For many of them, the shaving of pubic hair, enemas, the lithotomy position, pharmaceutical pain relief, and episiotomies were routine obstetrical procedures they experienced in hospital. Their husbands were not always allowed into labor and delivery rooms, and their newborn babies were often whisked away to nurseries and held to strict feeding schedules. Many of these routine procedures have since been shown to be of no obstetrical value. At best, they are convenient for physicians and nurses; at worst, they are the source of measurable harm to mother and infant (Davis-Floyd 1992; Hartmann et al. 2005; Thacker and Stroup 1999).

Many midwifery clients feel that what should be a natural continuity in knowledge and caring about childbirth between mother and daughter has been severed. Anna Lisa, for example, is a woman in her late thirties with three children—all born at home with the care of midwives. Before having her children she worked in the city as a fashion photographer, and now she stays home with her children in a house in the country. She told me that her mother had been "ethered" for the births of her first three children and had to fight to be allowed to stay awake for her fourth. Anna Lisa was close to her mother, but her mother couldn't tell her very much about labor and birth. Part of her satisfaction with midwifery care came from her sense that midwifery is a kind of maternal nurture and knowledge gained from having had children.

> I liked going to [my midwife] Gwen's house and her kids were running around and it was just really different. For the first two [of my babies, because it was before legislation] I also went to my doctor and the doctor kept the typical chart—you know the one I mean where they draw a little fundal height thing. And Gwen's appointments were more like "let's talk about breastfeeding, let's talk about feelings." I remember that I always felt way more confident about the baby's position after I left Gwen's place because it seemed to me that she was, like, really feeling where the baby was as opposed to the doctor. So it was almost like the doctor was the scientist and Gwen was like this "touchy-feely" person who was going to be there, like my mom, except my mom didn't know how to do it, so Gwen was going to come.

Furthermore, she felt that Gwen, as a mother of five, could truly empathize with her during labor and birth. As she describes it,

Gwen was very good at just kind of commiserating. Like if
she got the feeling that you needed your back rubbed and your
hair stroked, and if she thought that you weren't into physical
touching, then she would just be beside you and rock with you
and go, "Oh, yeah," in a low moan or, "That was good, that was
good." A little commiseration and a little encouragement.

Motherhood is seen by many midwives and women seeking their
care in Ontario to be an essential prerequisite for midwifery. Bridget,
who shared her "politically incorrect" opinion that all midwives
should be mothers, has five children. She also has two undergradu-
ate degrees—in music and French literature—and had not planned to
become a midwife. Rather, she describes being "called" to midwifery
through her personal experiences of pregnancy and motherhood.

Back then, it was a calling. It had to be a calling. We didn't
set out applying to a school. It was very traditional. It was the
natural work of women who had children, who felt a calling. We
saw what was happening, and we responded. I certainly didn't
think of it as a career.

Adding more detail about how her calling unfolded from her motherhood, Bridget continued.

Well, my first child was born in '74. We came home from France
and we wanted to have a home birth, and we realized there was
no one to attend a home birth, so we didn't get to have one. And
then the second one came three years later, and there was still
no one to attend a home birth even though we worked pretty
hard at that. It was just around the time when books were being
published and the movement was happening. I mean, none
of us knew that we were in a movement, we were just being
ourselves. So I found a family physician . . . who did home births
and we had a home birth! We met him quite regularly during
that time, and I sort of became a little bit of a resource for other
people. And I eventually started working with him. And then

a midwife moved to town a few months after [my second child] was born in '76, from Britain. It was just at the time when people were starting to get interested and [this midwife] . . . began to be asked. And around the same time I did some training to teach home birth preparation classes through the Association of Childbirth at Home. And then she asked me if I wanted to be her attendant . . . And it just sort of went from there . . .

Bridget identifies her midwifery calling as partly religious ("though not in any narrow sense"), partly "the natural work of women who had children," and also as a contribution to her community and society. She accepts this role regardless of remuneration and social recognition and in fact was one of the midwives who questioned the push for legislation to regulate midwifery in Ontario, fearing the loss of its principles. She notes with some disdain that she sometimes gets calls from young women interested in becoming midwives because the pay is so good or because it is trendy. Though Bridget is happy to be properly remunerated and recognized for her work, she believes she would have continued to practice regardless.

Motherhood and professional midwifery is a highly demanding combination. Full-time midwives work between sixty and eighty hours a week. Midwives regularly miss or are called away from important family events and holidays—birthdays, school plays, anniversaries, Christmas dinners. Reflecting on the enormous strain that midwifery can place on one's personal life, more than one midwife in my study ruefully called 1994—the first year of regulated midwifery in Ontario—"the year of the divorce."[10] Indeed midwives face a "caring dilemma," when, as workers, they have a duty to care for others which is promoted over their personal life and nonpaid work as partners and parents (Benoit and Heitlinger 1998). The pressure stems from a number of sources: midwives who believed strongly in continuity of care and thus made this one of the three clinical principles of the Ontario model of care, clients who demand a close relationship, and the increased administrative and clinical demands of working as regulated professionals within the health care system. Overall the relationship of the role of midwife to maternal nurture is complex. While one's personal experiences of pregnancy, birth, and motherhood can contribute to becoming a good midwife, the trend in Ontario is toward defining midwifery as a kind of wisdom, skill, and caring of which many are potentially capable.

Extending Care into the Community

Katherine is a midwife in her early forties living in a rural area in Ontario. The way that she became a midwife also began with motherhood.

> What happened to me is a story that you do hear in the caring professions—it comes from caring in some way in your own life and then extending that into your work life. [When I moved out of the city] there were not a lot of career opportunities. So I decided I'd start having my family, and the first thing I thought was important was to find a midwife. I quickly discovered there were less than five midwives at hand, and they were all in metropolitan Toronto or there were a couple in Kitchener or in Ottawa. But they were inaccessible to me. They couldn't travel to my home. So I became very committed to the movement of midwifery. I decided that if I really felt that midwifery was an essential component of my life while I was having my children, then other women must feel that way. But I wanted it to come to my community. I didn't want to have to move away. So I became committed to becoming a midwife. It sounds almost too grassroots in a way, but it did grow up exactly that way. I immediately became an advocate of breastfeeding in the community, and that's how I hooked up with [my practice partner]; [this kind of work] is very difficult to do as a single person in a community where the political will is against you.
>
> I also decided that I had to work politically in the city, where I knew [the HPLR] had called for submissions, and I knew that they always needed someone to type or to file papers. Generally, I knew that if I could support the movement, the chances for me of having a midwife for my next baby were much higher even if

they still weren't regulated. But I was absolutely positive when
I had that first baby that I knew midwives would be part of the
health care system here, and I never thought any other way. I
couldn't believe that my mother had me and my brother at home
years ago, and here I was wanting to do the same thing and I
couldn't even access it.

Determined to have midwifery in her own community for herself and for other women, Katherine sought out a local family physician—the very one that had delivered her—and tried to convince
him to attend the birth of her first baby at home. He initially refused.
With Katherine's urging, however, eventually this doctor started going to home births with her. There were a number of women in her
community who had home births in British Columbia who invited
Katherine along with the doctor to their births. As she describes it,
the doctor would sit off to the side letting Katherine and her practice
partner manage the labor and catch the baby. They worked with him
in the hospital, too—doing prenatal and labor support for all of his
first-time patients. This relationship with the friendly family physician
worked well for a time. Then, as Katherine describes it, "everything
got politically active and the community started closing down and not
wanting us labor supporting women." Even as she surmounted the
problem of her geographical isolation from urban centers where midwifery was more firmly established (two hundred kilometers away),
her local challenges began to multiply. Katherine faced a largely conservative medical community that was not ready for the changes that
midwifery would bring nor the challenge to the status quo that it
implied. Furthermore, she faced a situation of ongoing health care
restructuring that reduced medical services to rural areas of the province. Nevertheless, she and her practice partner persevered.

I work in rural Ontario. That's were I trained and grew up as
a midwife and it's very, very important . . . I just had a Danish
midwife visiting, and when she saw where I worked, she said
"How does it feel to be out here an hour from a hospital in
a snowstorm?" and I said "It feels great, just fine . . ." It's not

safety, you see, it's accessibility. For all of us [living in rural areas], if we have a heart attack, the chance of our survival is really minimal. And knowing that, we have chosen this quality of life. And then all around us the government closes hospitals—which really reduces our chances of survival more! But it really makes you say, "Well then, I want to take my own health care into my own hands. If you're telling me that all my services are going to be reduced then I feel safer—instead of traveling in the storm, trying to get to your hospital way up in [the nearest urban center] because you say that's where I ought to have my baby—I want trained providers to come to me . . . I recognize the risks of living here. I live with it everyday!" Farm women in particular feel that they are totally at that kind of risk all the time, and so are their children. So they just take control of it.

While she evokes her own experiences of birth and motherhood, what motivated Katherine to become a midwife was her vision of a rural community where people have access to safe birthing options that fit the context of their lives. It seems equally likely that Katherine could have chosen another profession that would have been compatible with such a vision, that midwifery is a means to an end, not necessarily the end in itself.

There is another detail in Katherine's story that speaks to the limits of the maternal nurture model for understanding her work as a midwife; that is, her need to draw the line between caring for her family and caring for her clients.

I only saw women in my home for a very short period of time when we were not regulated in the very early 1980s. I quickly discovered that to be in a profession where I was required to care so much that I couldn't share my family life as well. I couldn't have my clinic in my house. So my partner had the clinic in her house for almost five years. I don't know how she coped with it.

Putting the ideal of maternal nurture into practice can be hard on midwives, and Katherine was not the only midwife relieved to have her clinic out of her house. Many midwives welcomed the move to office spaces after regulation because it meant a clearer division between home and work, and also a stronger sense of being a "professional" (Sharpe 1998, 210). Such details speak to the limits of the idea of midwifery as maternal nurture and simultaneously to an important gender expectation that midwives have of women they care for, which would seem to run counter to the intimacy of maternal nurture. The ideal of an equal partnership between midwife and client which allows women to take responsibility for their own care is a key ingredient in women's feelings of empowerment through pregnancy and birth, and it is a clear gender expectation midwives have of the women in their care.[11]

Asta, a midwife in her early thirties, is unmarried, with no children. Midwifery combines her academic strengths and social interests. She holds a degree in human biology and undertook several years of midwifery apprenticeship in another province before enrolling in the MEP in Ontario and graduating with one of the first baccalaureate degrees in midwifery in Canada. She is not sure whether she will have children or not and does not see it as critically important to her chosen profession. For her, midwifery is about supporting women's choices. Yet she is strongly attached to midwifery as part of her identity; it is not just a job to her. While sharing many things with other midwives in terms of training and commitment to the profession, Asta has a clear vision of midwifery that does not involve the kind of natural selfless caring that is often associated with mothering. She related several stories to me about having to set boundaries for herself when clients sought too much intimacy with her or asked for advice about personal problems that did not even indirectly relate to their pregnancies (such as when to throw a birthday party for a difficult sister-in-law).

Though I did not expect midwifery in Ontario to share a close kinship with romanticized anthropological and popular descriptions that essentialize midwifery as maternal nurture, in asking the question, much has been revealed. Midwifery as maternal nurture is an idea that has been employed to contrast midwife-client relationships with stereotypically distant physician-patient relationships, and to contrast empirical hands-on learning with disembodied book learning. Midwifery knowledge and caring may be inspired and facilitated by personal experiences of labor, birth, and motherhood, but it does not depend upon it. Rather, midwifery knowledge, caring, and skill must be interpreted in the context of the intersection of interests that now produce midwifery in the province. First, nowhere in the official philosophy of informed choice, continuity of care, and choice of birth place is the idea of midwives as mothers first. Second, the knowledge, caring, and skill central to midwifery appears to be of a kind that any person is potentially capable of possessing or learning. Third, midwifery in Ontario is further distinguished from its historical and anthropological referents in that it is more clearly secular and politicized. As the stories of Katherine and Asta illustrate, midwifery is underpinned by interests, abilities, and concerns that go beyond motherhood to focus on supporting women's choices and to realize visions of what constitutes acceptable reproductive health care for women, such as accessible, informed choice and low-tech approaches. Furthermore, the kind of caring central to midwifery rests increasingly on politicized claims about gender—who women are and what they can do.

"Feminist Praxis"

Although midwifery challenges medical control, it does not challenge the traditional definition of women as mothers. Many supporters of the midwifery movement may hesitate to define its aims as feminist and make alliances with other movements working towards women's control of reproduction. (Van Wagner 1988, 117)

In the years since this observation was made, much has changed. Or perhaps only now, in the relative security of legislation, do midwives themselves (and those who study midwifery) feel they can represent midwifery in ways that deviate from the less-threatening association with the concerns of motherhood or in ways that are more explicitly feminist. From a feminist perspective, the idea that midwifery affirms and advocates a return to natural, selfless mothering as one of the central roles for women is problematic. Yet such an apparently essentializing move must be seen in the context of a contemporary midwifery ideology that radically reinterprets women as strong and capable in their roles as birthers, attendants, and mothers. The knowledge gained through childbearing and child rearing is seen as inherently valuable and, moreover, as a basis for women's consciousness raising and emancipation from biomedicine as a system of social control (Barrington 1985; Gaskin 1989). Scholars, too, have extolled the empowering potential of childbirth, birth attendance, and mothering within a contemporary midwifery framework. Notably, Barbara Katz Rothman has described midwifery as "feminist praxis" (1989).

Lisa is a midwife in her late thirties who has practiced in northern and southern Ontario. She explains that becoming a midwife occurred for her in the context of her interest and activism in women's health politics, including volunteer work as a counselor in an abortion clinic. Her pro-choice politics were at odds with what she found was an undercurrent of "pro-natalism and anti-choice thinking in midwifery."[12] Pointing out this political division within midwifery between pro-choice and anti-choice views on abortion was another indicator that the path to midwifery for her had led first through social activism. At the time she became interested in midwifery she was childless. As a feminist and women's health worker, Lisa felt that for women to achieve health they needed to have control over their own bodies. Midwifery fit into her vision of what constituted acceptable health care for women. She was motivated to become involved in midwifery because it offered reproductive choices for women.[13] In the mid-1980s Lisa joined a group of community midwives in her city who were organizing and lobbying for professionalization in the province. Only after several years of devoting one or two days a week of her time to this effort did she begin her clinical training to become a midwife. She now has a child, and while I cannot assume that it is irrelevant to her work, Lisa did not mention her own experience with childbirth and motherhood in any of our lengthy discussions about why she became a midwife or what midwifery means to her.

Student and aspiring midwives increasingly state their motivation to become midwives as rooted in social work and political activ-

ism and frequently have a great deal of volunteer experience in places
such as hospices, shelters for teenage mothers, and resource centers for
refugee women. Indeed, there is a sense among aspiring midwifery
students that to get a place in the Midwifery Education Program one
must demonstrate a commitment to social and political involvement,
as well as academic ability in the biological sciences. The maternal
nurture / ancient tradition / feminist activist strains of midwifery are
not irreconcilable. On the contrary, they are intertwined through a
formulation of gender in which women are strong and capable and
may know this power through their bodies in pregnancy, childbirth,
and motherhood, as well as through other experiences as apparently
disparate as living a rural life, engaging in social activism, or exploring feminist ideology through study.

Tradition as a Political Symbol

> There was a certain pioneering thing about it when we all
> started. There were risks. There were people who trusted us to
> be there at their births. They were also unusual, those women.
> They were doing something special too.
>   —Laura, Midwife

Closely related to the notion of midwifery as an extension of
motherhood experiences is the appealing portrayal of midwifery as an
ancient tradition—timeless, enduring, universal—found in both popular and scholarly accounts.[14] Early on in my fieldwork, my attention
was drawn to a brief vignette that still airs on television across Canada
entitled "Midwife: A Heritage Minute." This vignette portrays a
Canadian midwife who travels by horse-drawn sleigh and then by
snowshoes across a winter landscape to attend her neighbor in childbirth. In a log cabin lit by fire and lamplight, the midwife coaches the
woman through the last moments of labor and birth and then catches
the child as the woman's husband and other children look on. The
mother gives a cry of joy and relief, and we see the newborn baby
bathed in lamplight as the voiceover says, "Until well into this century most of us Canadians were born where we lived. And the only

professional hands guiding our arrival in the world were theirs: The Midwife." According to its promotional material, this vignette "dramatizes the importance and stature of the midwife in Canadian history: a skilled midwife risks the hazards of a rural winter to deliver a child on an isolated farm. The mother and father depend upon the midwife's calm skill, and the training she probably received from her own mother."[15]

This celebratory vignette presents a valorized image of traditional neighbor midwifery in Canadian history—hardy, wise, resourceful women making the best of things under difficult circumstances. On the one hand, it appears to simply document a piece of Canadian history. On the other hand, it might be read as a timely piece of public relations for the way it revalorizes traditional midwifery at precisely the historical moment when several Canadian provinces have moved to legalize midwifery after more than a century of official absence. As I have suggested in Chapter Two, the new midwifery in Canada has been strongly influenced by this particular historical image of midwifery and the trials it subsequently endured: denigration and near erasure at the hands of biomedicine, an alegal status throughout much of the twentieth century, and the generally wary and sometimes hostile relations between community midwives and formal health care providers over the last several decades as it reemerged. Indeed, the traditional neighbor midwife became iconic in the "recovery project" (Biggs 2004, 17) of professional midwifery, underpinning the sense of triumphal renaissance that was felt in 1994 when midwifery was officially recognized in Ontario. Closely linked to the iconic traditional midwife is the natural birth that she attends. The absence of biomedicine, the presence of the midwife's knowledge and skills, and the capable body of the birthing woman in a home setting are crystallized in the notion of the natural birth attended by a traditional, pre-demise Canadian midwife.

Despite the positive image it portrays, Maya, a midwife in my study, dislikes the Heritage Minute vignette. She thinks it perpetuates a mythical version of midwifery which conflicts with her own experience of being a young, urban-based midwife who carries a cell phone and drives an SUV. Yet she simultaneously expresses a sense of kinship with the pioneering spirit of traditional midwifery. Maya began her career in her late twenties by apprenticing with several midwives in her community and later went to El Paso, Texas, for a four-month residency in a private midwifery clinic there, receiving a permit to practice in the State of Texas. She was registered in Ontario in December 1993 with the first batch of midwives through the Michener Institute. Now in her late thirties, she runs a practice in the mid-sized Ontario town where she had always worked and lived. Maya's ambivalence about the Heritage Minute flags the problem that while contemporary midwifery's engagement with tradition has been made to appear self-evident in popular and scholarly accounts, it is, in fact, complex and contested.

Tradition, in its literal sense, refers to things passed down from one generation to the next—including knowledge, practices, and material objects. As theory in anthropology highlights, however, "culture" and "tradition" are best understood not as stable realities but as flexible human inventions of the present, as "on-going interpretation[s] of the past" (Handler and Linnekin 1984, 275). Moreover, a group's identification with tradition is often used as a rhetorical strategy in political struggles of the present (Hanson 1989) or as a "political symbol" (Keesing 1982) because calling something a tradition creates a sense of authenticity and ownership for the group making that claim. To understand tradition as invented does not invalidate its authenticity nor the right of the group or culture to claim it but rather draws analytical attention to the processes of its production and use. National, ethnic, cultural, and professional groups alike use culture and tradition to define themselves and, significantly, to distinguish themselves from other groups, as do social and political movements. How both positive and negative readings of traditional midwifery are employed in Canadian midwifery's professional and ideological struggles exemplify what Janice Boddy refers to as "managing tradition" (1995).

There is a sense among midwives and their supporters in Ontario that they have won a real victory not only in terms of gaining professional status but also of maintaining a philosophy of care and a scope of clinical practice that honors the essence of midwifery as a traditional practice of women helping women in childbirth.[16] Indeed the process to incorporate the very first group of midwives into the health care system in Ontario was known informally as the "granny-ing in" process. Many midwives identify strongly with the image of the traditional midwife as having qualities of sociality and caring, and they fear the loss of this aspect of tradition in the face of new bureaucratic and institutional demands brought on by regulation. Maya herself, while insistent that the public image of midwives needs updating, is wary of putting too much distance between contemporary midwifery and the idealized past.

> I don't ever want to see my practice get to the point where I am just checking off boxes and examining test results. I want to be able to continue to give that nurturing that I give . . . [Unfortunately] I don't see midwifery even lasting the way it was—taking time to make some bread for the mother while she's in labor, or comb her hair, or nurture her. I see it becoming very professionalized and losing some of those old doula kind of skills, that mothering kind of skill.[17] And that is because we don't have the time . . . I see midwifery changing, and as hard as we fight to have it not change from that romantic thing of going out in the middle of the night—how can it not? We have cell phones and fax machines and pagers and a heavy caseload and papers and committees and [we are] doing fifteen jobs at once and wearing eighteen different hats.

Midwives in Ontario also remember a certain clinical autonomy that came with being outside the mainstream health care system. Maya herself notes how bureaucratic obligations now impinge upon these "traditional" forms of caring for women in labor. Another midwife in Maya's area ruefully refers to her work since legislation as "with chart" rather than "with woman," referring to the mounds of paperwork now required, especially when she attends deliveries in the hospital. Other midwives describe the loss of ability to exercise a special kind of clinical judgment or authoritative knowledge (Jordan 1993), sometimes expressed as intuition.

Lillian, for example, is a midwife in rural practice who has worked in northern Ontario most of her career. She typifies in many ways the combination of a nursing background, formal midwifery training at a foreign institution, and home birth apprenticeship. She was in favor of professionalization because it offers the public greater access to midwives and greater assurance of their qualifications. At the same time, she strains under some of the new professional standards.

> There was a certain freedom before midwifery was incorporated into the system, in the sense that although we had a very strong professional association that had very well-defined standards of practice, the midwives were less bound by medical standards than we are now . . . As people outside of the system, we could have a little bit more leeway, we could be a little bit more flexible in terms of what this individual woman needs instead of being bound by the medical standard. Now we are a lot more caught into the system. For example, there are circumstance where I may not be able to do what I think is best because I am bound by medical standards.

Another way in which midwives fear the loss of tradition is through the standardization of midwifery education, which some feel will further erode the connection of midwifery to the historical past. They also fear a loss of connection with the more recent past of midwifery as a social movement—a radical challenge to the status quo that honed its identity and ideals through the experience of practicing outside the system—a structural location conceptually tied to notions of traditional midwifery and to midwifery's critique of medicalization. These sentiments are captured well in the words of Laura, a midwife mentioned in Chapter Two, who was largely self-trained and practiced for thirteen years in Ontario before legislation.

> Yes, one can feel proud that one has these skills and that one can order medication and perform certain procedures. These are certainly skills that I'm glad I have. But in terms of my connection with tradition, I feel sad about certain things because I see myself going in that other direction more and more.

Especially those [student midwives] who have no background in the tradition of midwifery before legislation, they will not understand its value. They will know nothing of it. Right now it's a matter of degrees. Right now the majority of us practicing have that experience. And then you are going to have the midwifery students who, say, had a midwife before legislation or were childbirth educators before legislation—something. They will have some knowledge about it. And then eventually it's all going to disappear. There is going to be nobody who has any experience about what that was. They will only have heard about it in class or whatever, and you see that now.

The identification of contemporary midwifery with a strong social and cultural tradition and system of non-medical authoritative knowledge is what draws many women to choose midwifery care in Ontario today. Traditional midwifery also implies certain gendered characteristics of birthing women as strong and capable which counteract notions of birthing women as incapable and weak, and of birth as something that women *do*, rather than as something that *happens to* women. Furthermore, the friends and neighbors whom traditional midwives attended in Canada were perceived as the social equals of their midwives. Midwifery in Ontario continues to strive to reproduce this egalitarian dynamic between midwives and the women they attend—though it can be challenging to do so. Thus, important political strategies are embedded in this positive engagement with tradition. Midwives hold on to an identification with traditional midwifery that stands in opposition to the bureaucratization and scientization of their knowledge and the hierarchy of doctor-patient relationships.

Sociologist Cecilia Benoit suggests that while a certain critical nostalgia "can be helpful in challenging the many negative aspects of medically dominated maternity care, the accompanying bias towards pre-modern midwifery remains problematic" (1991, 92). Aware of this pitfall, midwives speak of the need to strike a balance between those aspects of their work stereotypically associated with either tradition or modern medicine. Martina, another rural midwife, tells me

My great-grandmother was a midwife . . . so I sort of have this idea that there is still a bit of that in my blood. But at the same time—I mean, we don't just get called during labor—it's much more clinical. We are doing blood work that my grandmother wouldn't have done and more lab work and tests. But I want to hold on to some of that. I don't want to become a techno midwife. It's not what I want to do at all. It doesn't mean that we don't use technology or are not willing to—we certainly do, all the time. But I think that one thing that attracts women to midwives and certainly attracts women to become midwives is that sense of the neighbor, the friend, having a cup of tea. It is more friendly; you've got time to spend time with women.

Important political strategies are embedded in more negative readings of traditional midwifery as well. Sonja, whom I introduced earlier, is a midwife in her mid-forties with three children. She is largely self-taught and has worked in her rural community for more than ten years. Perhaps because of her rural location, she is not so nostalgic about tradition if it means isolation from the modern health care system. She suggests that contemporary midwifery in Ontario should be careful to distinguish itself from traditional midwifery in some particular ways.

In a Third-World country or the far North if you can't possibly get to a hospital within a reasonable time, you might as well stay where you are and make the best of things; you can decide that these are the limits of what we can do and just sort of hope for the best. In this part of the country where we have access to hospitals, we have access to emergency service, we have access to lots of technology; there isn't a defensible way to not use it. (There are) the parts of the traditional holistic approach that we can't continue on with, or refuse to give up—we can't just sit there and watch things happen. We have to intervene . . . we can't step back and decide that we'll go back to the way things were at the turn of the century when we just sort of let nature take its course.

While her portraits of midwifery in "a Third-World country" or "the far North" may be subjective, the point is that Sonja's position rejects the perceived naturalism and fatalism associated with traditional midwifery. She welcomes the chance to "move midwifery into the twenty-first century." It is an important, if somewhat polarizing, critique of tradition as a barrier to progress which falls clearly within feminist strategies to selectively embrace technology as a route to women's empowerment, harnessing it for their own ends (Firestone 1972; Haraway 1991; Lock and Kaufert 1998; Sawicki 1991).[18]

In a similar vein to this discussion, sociologist Beth Rushing has looked at Canadian and U.S. independent midwives' uses of ideology, which she defines as "a set of beliefs by which a social group makes sense of its environment and which these groups manipulate in order to project images of themselves" (1993, 47) and which she understands as "on-going social processes that are not fixed but are shaped also by the uses to which they are put" (1993, 47). Her definition of ideology in the context of health professions and the way they pursue "occupational power" is similar to anthropological definitions of tradition and culture as they are used in analyses of cultural identity formation and practice. Rushing observes that in public representations of midwifery in particular, science and feminism are the two ideologies most often used as legitimating strategies, while other important ideologies remain more in the background. The ambivalence regarding tradition in Ontario speaks to the need to juggle these (sometimes apparently competing) ideological associations for strategic purposes in public representations with the more personal views and feelings of midwives and midwifery clients that I discuss here. Martina's ambivalence about tradition, for example, is clearly bound up with the struggle to gain and maintain access to institutional spaces and modern medical technology; a struggle that figured prominently in the project to gain professional status for midwives and choices for birthing women. How midwives and their clients avail themselves of medical technology, and what they make of it, is a key component of the new midwifery in Ontario, which I take up in more detail in Chapter 4.

One of the most vivid midwifery stories from my fieldwork was told by rural midwife Katherine. I had been to visit her practice earlier in the year and had met and interviewed several of her clients. Our last conversation, in contrast, took place in the lobby of a hotel where she had been staying while she was in the city for some meetings. I asked for her thoughts on traditional midwifery. How close did she feel to that image? What value did she attach to it? "I certainly can say that I get to play the pioneer a lot," she responded, echoing the sentiments and stories of many other midwives in the province. "I often do births with no phones and no power, and in places where we have to stoke the stove ourselves." One particularly memorable night she was called to a home birth during a severe snowstorm. The roads were closed. Katherine drove her car as far as she could and then skied the rest of the way to the house, carrying all her equipment on her back. "I was the only help [this woman] had! So I went in on my skis and was not fearful at all. I just did the pioneer thing." The birth went smoothly, and mother and baby were fine.

This midwifery story is so compelling because it evokes a Canadian national identity rooted in the histories of European settlement: the pioneering spirit of strong and capable men and women together against the elements of weather and isolation. In this way, midwifery is ideal Heritage Minute material. Even as I sat across from Katherine, soaking up the images of this marvelous story, she moved on quickly to say that midwifery is not really about such memorable exceptions, nor it is about making the best of things in difficult or dire circumstances. The new midwifery, she insists, is about making a unique model of low-intervention, woman-centered maternity care work in a practice with other midwives and in a larger network of trained professionals and public health services. Of the emergence of midwifery and its foray into the public system in the late twentieth century, Katherine carefully extends the familiar metaphor, concluding: "We truly are pioneering for women's health."

If a new minute-long vignette about midwifery in Canada were to be made, Katherine would like to see a home birth scene that includes two midwives and their clinical gear. In Maya's version, the midwife would be under forty and not necessarily a mother. This time the midwife would get a phone call or her pager would go off. "There's no little girl knocking at her log cabin door. And she would take off in her four-wheel drive in a snowstorm and she would do some pretty horrible roads out there. And she would be doing a home birth; maybe there's a fire going, but there could be also beautiful classical music in the background."

Looking to the history of midwifery in this country or to birthing practices in other cultures in search of an authentic traditional midwifery tends not to provide certainties about how things once were or how they should be. Rather, my attention to tradition as a political symbol highlights midwives' agency in the cultural (re)construction of their work, as well as the contributions of birthing women. As we have seen, midwives in Ontario imagine and manage tradition with some ambivalence. They draw positive connections between themselves and traditional midwives in terms of the personalized, patient, continuous, and low-tech care they offer their clients. This engagement with tradition works to maintain symbolic and practical links to midwifery as a social movement in the 1970s and 1980s which explicitly employed ideas of tradition as a political symbol to define itself in opposition to biomedicine, to restore the definition of birth as a natural event that could take place in the home, and to reinvent women as competent birthers and attendants. Meanwhile, midwives are careful to distance themselves from certain negative and fatalistic aspects of tradition in order to establish their status as legitimate professionals in the formal health care system, maintain access to modern technology and institutions, and secure choices for birthing women. Thus the new midwifery in Ontario is selective and strategic in its association with tradition, taking into account the context of its present-day location and concerns. While my analytical approach breaks up the possibility of a genuine traditional midwifery to which we might all refer, it does not necessarily break up the power of tradition as a political symbol. Being part of midwifery tradition or birth culture will continue to provide for midwives and their clients a sense of authenticity and ownership over this particular model of care because of its power to mark as "midwifery" those clinical practices, places, and ways of caring for pregnant and birthing women that differ from mainstream medical care.[19]

Midwifery and the Romance of Resistance

Reading midwifery as resistance is another compelling approach to analyzing this cultural system. Anthropologists have shown how midwives and birthing women in diverse cultural and historical contexts have maneuvered under conditions of gender oppression, colonialism, capitalist penetration, development, and medical hegemony, and how they interpret, appropriate, and resist centralizing, medicalizing forces. Molly Dougherty (1978), for example, describes how granny midwives in the southern United States, despite state regulations that prohibit certain social and ritual practices, and despite the routine and vocal objections of public health nurses, continue to rely on prayer and magical practices at home births—away from the disciplining gaze of biomedicine and the state.[20] Denise Roth Allen (2004) describes how village women in Tanzania continue to utilize the local midwife rather than face a cold and patronizing medical clinic. Brian Burtch (1994) describes community midwifery in the interior of British Columbia in the 1980s as a form of civil disobedience. Anthropologists have rightly treated such activities as resistance because their actions interrupt and alter the forces of biomedical expansion and state intervention.[21] Scholars studying midwifery, however, have also shown a tendency to "romanticize resistance" (Abu-Lughod 1990a). Can professional midwifery in Ontario still be read as resistance, given its new social and political relations as a profession with biomedicine and the state? Or has midwifery been co-opted and ceased to be a social movement?

Certainly, much has changed for midwives and their clients in Ontario in the past ten years. As a regulated profession and publicly funded maternity care service, midwifery is now part of the very social and political institutions that it challenged and opposed for many years. Indeed, the midwifery community itself made a case against regulated midwifery on the basis that professionalization would alter the fundamentals of midwifery practice and thus destroy its status as a social movement resisting medicalization and state surveillance of women's bodies. Midwife and scholar Betty Anne Daviss argues that "the radical flank" is now largely missing from professional midwifery

(2001, 82). Below, I take up several concerns and critiques about the erosion of midwifery's ability to effectively maintain its resistance to medicalized childbirth.

But first, a little theory. In anthropology it used to be that issues of conflict and acts of resistance and protest were treated seriously only when they were collective and large scale, but recent theory and ethnographic case studies have demonstrated the importance of looking at resistance when it is individual and particularistic (Abu-Lughod 1990a; Comaroff 1985; Scheper-Hughes and Lock 1991). Abu-Lughod notes new concern with smaller, less likely forms of local resistance not necessarily tied to the overthrow of political or ideological system (1990, 41); indeed she urges us to look at forms for resistance everywhere—especially in the discourses of body, health, and gender—and to treat them as "non-trivial." Yet Abu-Lughod cautions against reading all forms of resistance as signs of human freedom and suggests that they tell us rather about "forms of power and how people are caught up in them" (1990, 42). In other words, resistance does not erase power but serves as evidence of it and exists simultaneously with it (Foucault 1980a, 95–96).

Jutta Mason, a long-time midwifery supporter and critic of professionalization in Ontario, warned in an essay "The Trouble with Licensing Midwives" (1990), that allowing the state to regulate midwives would fundamentally alter the relationship between the midwife and the women she attended, and would shift power in decision making away from birthing women. Ivy Lynn Bourgeault (2006) in her study of the process and outcome of the incorporation of midwifery in Ontario concludes that new state and medical constraints on midwives have served to distance them from their clients and to wear away the ideal of the equal partnership around which midwifery was built and flourished. Whereas midwifery used to be regulated by birthing women in negotiation with their midwife caregivers, it is now, Bourgeault argues, regulated by a professional body that represents midwives. The midwife–client relationship is a great deal more complicated than either the ideal of the equal partnership or the hierarchical physician–client relationship against which it is posed. While

it is true that many things have changed since legislation which impinge upon the midwife-client relationship, the nature, degree, and
evaluation of these changes are contested.

The charge that professionalization has created an un-midwifery-
like distance between midwife and client relies to some extent on
an idealized relationship between midwives and birthing women that
existed before regulation. The ideal of the equal partnership model of
midwifery, in turn, is predicated to some extent on the "ideal client"
of the past. Prior to legislation, women and their partners paid out of
pocket for midwifery services—usually in the range of eight hundred
to one thousand dollars. Clients of the past were repeatedly described
to me as "very committed" to healthy lifestyles, home birth, mothering, and alternative lifestyles. Midwife Sonja describes the changes in
her rural catchment area since the integration of midwifery into the
public health care system:

> People who paid for their care prior to legislation were pretty
> committed. People who wanted home births were in a category
> of commitment. [They were] committed to taking whatever
> happened in their care quite seriously, to taking responsibility
> for that, and so they were comfortable paying for their care
> outside the system, making whatever extra arrangements they
> had to in order to have the birth that they wanted, and paying
> for it. A lot of them were very well educated already and highly
> politicized. Some already were more "out there" as far as the
> kinds of holistic and natural approaches they were willing to go
> along with and the amount of technology they would allow in
> their care. That picture—no matter what kind of socioeconomic
> or education background they were coming from—that sort of
> describes most of the people prior to legislation . . . Once people
> could have midwives in the hospital and midwives paid for by
> the provincial government, you know, that opened the door to
> a large group of people who we wouldn't otherwise have seen
> . . . Now we have people who smoke, people who drink, people
> who want midwifery care because they don't think they want

to have doctor care, because they aren't comfortable with them. They are sort of coming for less clear reasons—like, their cousin told them, or their sister had one and they think that maybe it's a good idea, but they don't have any philosophical background. I mean, what do they think a midwife is? I have had to actually ask a couple of clients when we've run up against some barriers: why do you want midwifery care anyway? So, there has been a shift in clientele.

As Sonja describes, the consumer movement advocating for choices in childbirth that went hand in hand with midwifery as a social movement and a professionalization movement was overwhelmingly comprised of highly committed, well-educated, white, middleclass women. The incorporation of midwifery into the health care system has begun to fulfill the promise of accessibility to a wider clientele. Women's reasons for seeking midwifery care are also changing and sometimes diverge from what midwives themselves desire and expect. This has posed some challenges. Midwives lament that many women now choose midwifery care without knowing anything about midwifery as a social and political movement or the clinical practices that arose from midwifery's organized challenge to the biomedicalization of pregnancy. It represents to them a kind of decontextualized use of their services: choosing midwifery because you get longer appointments, home visits, continuity of care, a greater degree of emotional engagement and so on, but without understanding or believing in the struggle of midwifery as a feminist social movement. I have heard it called the "midwifery spritzer" or "midwifery à la mode."

Midwife Lillian describes the clientele in her large rural catchment area as ranging from rural farm women to professional women commuting into the city, to students, to teenagers. Her practice also serves the Amish and Mennonite communities. Lillian, however, meets this post-legislation diversity with a sense of challenge.

The idea of an ideal client makes no sense to me at all. It seems to me that a woman who is a smoker would benefit more from midwifery care because we would have an opportunity to be in discussion with her, to help her to cut down or quit. I mean, I can see, potentially, screening somebody out of a home birth if she was a smoker or if there was concern about the size of the baby. But I don't think it's really ethical, selecting someone on other than clinical criteria.

Lillian believes that most women she sees are seeking similar things, even though some may lack the overtly politicized outlook of most of the pre-legislation clients. But Lillian rises to the challenge of this sometimes "uneasy partnership" (Benoit 1987).

It's a challenge, but it's also what makes it interesting. I mean if I only ever saw women who ate health food and didn't smoke and were totally healthy, I would be missing a lot of learning opportunities as a midwife. I certainly want to give good care to my clients, but I also have needs in terms of what I want to get out of my profession; I want to be stimulated and challenged and continue to learn! And I think that I learn something from every birth that I attend—every client.

Though an increasing number of midwifery clients do not see their engagement with midwifery as overtly political—either as an act of resistance against the hierarchical doctor-patient relationship in mainstream maternity care or against the system and authoritative knowledge claims of medicine itself—we should not be too quick to dismiss "midwifery à la mode" as an entirely apolitical phenomenon. Women who choose midwifery care without the commitment to and understanding of it as a social and political project are part of midwifery in Ontario, too. And most have been made (sometimes painfully) aware that midwifery is still a statistically marginal, frequently misunderstood choice. By choosing midwifery (and also by participating in my study) even the midwifery à la mode clients are transgressing mainstream norms and boundaries, resisting the status quo, and creating counterstories and counterexperiences to the medical management of childbirth.

Embodied Politics

From a feminist perspective, theorizing midwifery used to be a lot easier: midwifery stood as the opposite of biomedical birth in the hospital. Participating in midwifery was an act of resistance to state intervention, to the medicalization, institutionalization, and even secularization of birth.[22] Recent theorizations of midwifery in the social sciences as hybrid have been helpful to expand beyond such oppositional readings. Sociologist Cecilia Benoit, for example, offers a portrait of midwifery in Newfoundland and Labrador which carefully avoids the temptation to romanticizing midwifery in this unique setting of far-flung outports and fishing villages (1991). Rather, she paints a complex picture of midwifery that includes stories of hardship, courage, commitment, and caring—quintessentially traditional—but also documents the changing relationship of midwives to biomedicine and the health care system. Sociologist Brian Burtch offers a similarly nuanced portrait of community midwifery in southern British Columbia in the mid-1980s—a movement of relatively young, urban or semi-urban, middle-class, literate, and well-educated women. On the one hand, Burtch clearly views the development of community midwifery in British Columbia as a form of civil disobedience, resisting statist ideology, circumventing authority and fostering "ideologies that emphasize women's power in childbirth and the privacy of the family sphere" (1988, 351). On the other hand, he observes that midwifery in BC is also clearly linked to science and formal institutional training. Midwifery is a hybrid, he concludes (1988, 365). Similarly, Davis-Floyd and Davis (1997) describe midwives in North America, as well as other parts of the world, as postmodern—an appellation that defines midwives as "articulate defenders of traditional ways as well as creative inventors of systems of mutual accommodation" who blend modern technology, scientific evidence, and institutions (1997, 242).

Many scholars have written of the appeal of hybridity in terms of its ability to dispel essentialisms and move away from the fetishization of discrete and timeless cultural systems so characteristic of classic anthropology. Others, however, caution against using hybridity as an all-purpose antidote to essentialism. Nicholas Thomas, for example, argues that "hybridity and similar concepts" can, in fact, reify old essentialisms, especially when thought of as some sort of perfect blending between two hitherto discrete cultural forms or times or places. Further, he suggests that if hybridity is understood as a stage—"a final step of progress from the past to the contemporary world"—then "it can be understood in an evaluative way which then reifies and affirms the distance between ancient and modern in an evolutionary sense" (1996, 9). In approaching an analysis of midwifery, this is something to be avoided. Like all identities—and scholarly analyses of them— the hybridity label is about "the efforts of value creation and political transformation" (Thomas 1996, 11) not unlike the essentialisms that it is said to combine. One more midwifery narrative moves us away from settling easily on hybridity or postmodernity—to the extent that these terms imply a kind of seamless blending of two certainties of time or place or ideological orientation—as a final analysis to something that is perhaps less stable but can take into account the contingencies of embodiment.

On a particularly clear and cold winter day, I drove north several hours to meet with two women who had had midwifery care, Sarah and Petra. We met at Sarah's home—a farmhouse perched on a hill overlooking a river valley. Not yet thirty years old, Sarah was already the mother of four—three girls born in hospital with physician care, and a boy—her "midwife birth"—born at home. At the time we met, she was pregnant with her fifth child and was planning another home birth with midwives. Petra is in her mid-forties with two children, three and seven, both born at home with midwives (one before and one just after regulation). Toward the end of our afternoon of conversation and food, I asked them if they consider themselves to be part of something beyond their personal experiences. Sarah responded,

> At the time I had my first two, I really didn't know anything about alternative methods. My father-in-law is a family doctor. I got in touch with the La Leche League, and that was a good way for me to meet women who were home with children. La Leche League was the first thing I did about making a statement about my parenting and what was important to me as a woman.

And from their library I started reading a lot about alternatives and started questioning how I had been cared for in the hospital. I started to think about how to have the birth I wanted—even with an obstetrician. But I didn't think at that time even about using a midwife, but more just about being my own advocate in the hospital.

From what she had already told me I knew that her decision to have a midwife and a home birth was a difficult one. Her story was not unremarkable in rural Ontario at a time when over 97 percent of women gave birth in hospitals with physician care. Her story is more remarkable for the fact that two years before the birth of her "midwife baby" at home, Sarah supported a close friend in her decision to have a home birth with midwifery care. Her friend's baby was delivered after a lengthy labor but failed to breathe on his own and died several hours later in hospital. Sarah had supported her friend all through her pregnancy and had even been with her at her home for a time during the labor to offer food and encouragement. She had also appeared at the inquest into the baby's death. This event occurred in 1990 on the eve of midwifery legalization, and the publicity and controversy surrounding it had been intense. Despite her closeness to this traumatic event and its aftermath, or perhaps because of it, and despite living in a community where the reception to midwifery remains somewhat hostile, the baby's death and the inquest that followed had the effect of politicizing her. Through it, she said, "I got to see how midwifery was working and how it was evolving." Sarah chose midwifery care for her fourth child and delivered at home. She is also planning a home birth for her fifth baby. This rather long exchange below between myself, Sarah, and her neighbor Petra, draws out her convictions about midwifery in the face of such complex circumstances.

Sarah: I think if there was no midwifery in Ontario, there would be. I mean, I think that it came to be because women were feeling like—you put some thought into the decisions that you are making. You don't just accept something because it's the status quo. You want things to be more natural. You are doing something that is better for your child. It's also about being confident in your femininity to breastfeed, that you don't see yourself as only a sexual image. There is a sort of wholeness to being a woman . . . [It is] a kind of confidence in yourself, the naturalness of it.

Petra: But it's not easy. I used to say, "Birth is not a pastel experience," because I hate this pastel idea of motherhood you know? It's purple and red and throbbing! It's very primal.

Sarah: Oh, yeah. I think that midwifery really supports those ideas; those are the kind of ideas that midwives have. They have faith in women. I mean they really have faith in women! [They say] "You have the ability to do this and I have faith in you."

Petra: Yes that's right. But I was worried that [with regulation] it might be regulating something that was occurring naturally anyway. Something that would occur no matter what the government said.

Sarah: Well, I think that the women involved in midwifery in Ontario were able to spearhead those kinds of feelings among women. That death on Toronto Island could have resulted in the opposite happening—it could have resulted in midwifery being illegal and midwives being charged with criminal offenses. And I think that if that had happened women would still seek out alternatives. I think there would still be a lot of women and a lot of families—not just women but fathers too—who would still seek out that kind of care for their pregnancies, for their births.

MM: Does it have anything to do with feminism?

Sarah: Yeah.

Petra: I think so. And activism in general. People knew how to mobilize and organize. In the early 1980s, I had some friends who were involved in the first "suck-in" at the Manulife Centre. (Laughter). I just thought "Oh! They are going to a suck-in!" and I didn't have any children or anything like that, but I thought those things are happening in Toronto. Well, I

guess Toronto is maybe a site [for activism] because it is a large
city and university town.[23]

Sarah: I don't remember the details of that [particular
demonstration], but I do remember these protests of women
nursing in local malls [which started] from a certain woman
being asked to leave and being told that she was offending
others.

Sarah and Petra see midwifery as having a "natural" origin, as
arising out of women's deeply personal experiences of pregnancy
and birth. At the same time, they position themselves within midwifery as a social movement through their own experiences in local and extralocal contexts—La Leche League meetings, demonstra-
tions in local malls, and "suck-ins" in downtown Toronto. For Sarah
and Petra, midwifery involves active organized resistance and the
pragmatic choices of women in local and personal contexts. Oddly
enough, Sarah's paradoxical assertion that "if there was no midwifery
in Ontario, there would be," I had heard several times before. Sometimes it was uttered dreamily, as if midwifery were an emotion that
could be masked but never truly suppressed. Indeed, two coroners'
inquests into infant deaths at midwifery-attended home births in the
1980s recommended that midwifery be implemented precisely because
they knew that midwifery and home birth would continue, regardless of legal measures to prevent it or even to criminalize it. There is a
hint too, in this sentiment, that midwifery—because it believes in and
supports the power of women to carry and give birth to children, because it is an embodied power—is something so wild that it will never
be tamed. Indeed, there are more than a few midwives and women in
Ontario who believe that midwifery should never have been regulated
and that professional midwifery is not real midwifery at all.[24]

Sarah and Petra believe, as do many other women and midwives,
that it was inevitable that some women took maternity care into their
own hands by giving birth at home, or by becoming midwives. It is
not simply that midwifery is an irrepressible tradition—because midwifery is practiced many different ways around the world—but that
a kind of embodied knowledge—not instinct but rather a culturally

embodied knowledge of the possibilities of who women are and what they can do—is *available* in pregnancy and childbirth and can give rise to a political consciousness when denied. Midwife Laura concurs.

> I think that there always have been women at all times who have very much wanted to be at home for their births, so it will go on as an underground thing if it doesn't go on as a fully approved thing. It will probably go in cycles—like in England, where they have midwifery, but in some areas they are not doing home birth, so people just say, "Well, then, we'll do it on our own." I think in one case a father even got arrested! So you have that sort of thing happening because you will always have people feeling this way; it may go underground, but it will always exist.
>
> It is so interesting to me to see the women who see us, who are just so sure about what they want to do—this gut feeling about what is right about giving birth. And even people who might be seen as higher risk—we all have had people who are just so dead set against the hospital. I don't know what it is that keeps that always there . . . For instance, [my colleague] had a client who had a couple of C-sections and had high blood pressure who signed herself out of the hospital . . . And when I see these women who are so convinced that they are right, I think, "They probably are!" There are also people who from a very religious or philosophical point of view are very "Well, whatever happens is meant to be," and they are prepared to deal with what happens . . . And there are always people who will be like that.

What is Midwifery?

Midwifery in Ontario is more than an extension of maternal nurture or simply the reemergence of an ancient tradition. Midwifery in Ontario is not only a radical and sophisticated feminist critique of the medicalization and institutionalization of pregnancy and of birth, but now mingles with the very modalities and places it once symbolically opposed (biomedicine, its institutions, and technologies.) Having won the struggle to be recognized by the province as a health profession, midwifery emerged from the margins with a clearly delineated scope of practice and was integrated into the formal health care system. But the struggle to create midwifery and also to define it is not won in legislation and legal definitions. And while I seem to be suggesting that we leave such labels as traditional, maternal, resistance, and even hybridity behind, midwifery continues to give meaning to childbirth through these powerful idioms of nature, tradition, home, and women's empowerment. Midwives and birthing women give meaning to and experience midwifery politically, pragmatically, instinctually, according to their own understandings and needs. Kirin Narayan's notion of the "enactment of hybridity" (1997) is fitting for contemporary midwifery in Ontario in that it gives the sense of midwifery not just as a professional or political identity but also as an activity that takes place within a field of power relations. That is, midwives and their clients in Ontario are actively producing midwifery in the context of a shifting set of social, political, and clinical relationships—innovating, inventing, and reinventing the profession of midwifery itself, as well as the experience of midwifery. This idea of midwifery as continually enacted on public and private stages, as processual, might also be used to expand the appealing idea of midwifery as postmodern, again injecting into this concept a measure of uncertainty and change and even intimacy.

In the chapters that follow, I narrow my focus to the topic of the discursive constructions and performances of the body within the wider structural and analytical fields that I have been mapping here. I hope to show that the relevance of this academic discussion of midwifery ideology and identity has implications in clinical practice. How midwives and their clients define the new midwifery in Canada informs the care that midwives provide, the knowledge that gets to count, and, ultimately, the gendered identities of women as birth attendants and the embodied experiences of women as birthers. For central to midwifery, however it is defined, are ideological and practical claims about gender—who women are and what they can do. At the heart of midwifery in Ontario is a campaign to reconfigure women's gendered identities as competent birthers and attendants.

CHAPTER FOUR

Natural Births and Gender Expectations

I think that natural is a stupid word. What does it mean in this society? I just wanted to have my birth. You know what I mean? I wanted to be the one who was making the decisions, or we were making the decisions. I didn't want to have a "natural" birth. I'm sure all of [my midwife's] clients would gladly use the hospital if they thought that their baby would die otherwise. I mean, we don't live in the hills. I just wanted to be able to trust myself in the experience of being pregnant and the experience of giving birth, and I want to now be able to do that with raising my children. (Leigh, 36, midwifery client)

THE NOTION OF NATURAL birth has long been used as a rhetorical strategy to counter the predominant biomedical or "technocratic" (Davis-Floyd 1994) model of the pregnant and birthing body as inherently problematic and potentially dangerous to the fetus. Midwives, birthing women, and women's health writers and activists have often appealed to the authority of nature as a legitimizing basis for midwifery ideals and clinical practices. In the new midwifery in Canada, natural birth is an idiom for what midwives clinically refer to as normal birth and, as such, carries a kind of cultural weight that goes beyond this latter term. From the perspective of anthropology and feminist theory, the nostalgic desire for birth as a natural event that takes place in the home, however compelling and strategic, is problematic. While in other realms of anthropological inquiry—kinship, medicine, gender, and nationalism—nature has been approached as a cultural construction, it has not been fully problematized in scholarly analyses of midwifery and childbirth. That such a notion should persist is not surprising, given the close relationship between midwifery scholarship and advocacy in the area of childbirth reform that I discussed in Chapter 1. Yet given the development of feminist theory and practice beyond such essentialisms—even strategic essentialisms (Spivak 1993)—it is perhaps time to illuminate just what it means.

Does midwifery in Ontario claim to have discovered or rediscovered the true nature of women's bodies and the natural facts of pregnancy and birth? Superficially, this might appear to be the case. When asked directly about natural birth, midwives and the birthing women they attend respond in predictable ways: "It means drug free"; "It means no interventions"; "It means non-medicalized, the opposite of a hospital birth." When probed, however, or approached through other issues, the question of what constitutes natural birth begins to reveal some unexpected dimensions. In this chapter I explore the discursive constructions and performances of the "natural" pregnant and birthing body within the wider structural and analytical fields of contemporary midwifery in Canada which I have been mapping in the previous chapters.[1] My specific focus is on the ideological and practical claims about gender—what I am calling gender expectations—inherent within the midwifery ideal of natural birth.

Part of the theoretical basis for this analysis lies with critical-interpretive theory in medical anthropology which posits that "all knowledge relating to the body, health and illness is culturally constructed, negotiated, and renegotiated in a dynamic process through time and space" (Lock and Scheper-Hughes 1990, 49). Scholars have demonstrated persuasively how scientific knowledge about reproduction through the ages has been embedded in concepts and practices already on hand, cultural notions about the true nature of men and women embedded in power hierarchies manifested as institutionalized knowledge and practices concerning the female body (Duden 1987; Gallagher and Laqueur 1987; Martin 1991; Oudshoorn 1994; Tuana

1989). Feminist theorists of the body have drawn on Foucault's concept of "biopower" to understand the history of women's bodies as products of the same disciplinary power/knowledge regimes that we see located within institutions such as hospitals, clinics, schools, and prisons (1975, 1977). Specifically, women's bodies have been scientifically constructed as essentially faulty; their reproductive bodies as potentially dangerous to babies; childbirth as so fraught with danger as to be unthinkable without biomedical surveillance and intervention.

Indeed, these "facts" of reproduction have worked to *naturalize* gender inequality and ideas of women as weak and incompetent and in need of male control and instruction (Yanagisako and Delaney 1995, 16). Feminist accounts of modern biomedical maternity care specifically document the negative impact of medicalization on women's bodies from birth to death. Davis-Floyd's term "technocratic birth" describes the constellation of ideas and institutional and clinical practices that characterize modern obstetrical medicine (1994) and which alienates women from their bodies, fragments the potential wholeness of the birth experience, and commodifies women and babies (Corea 1985; Martin 1987; Rothman 1982). One of the political goals of feminist scholarship on the gendered body has been to expose such layers of signification on the body built up by the regulatory and self-regulatory practices of culture and modern power. And for the past several decades, as science has continued to discover the "natural facts" of the female body, interested scholars have continued to expose these facts as cultural constructions. One could argue that the task of midwifery shares some similarities with this scholarly effort in terms of the desire to peel away the fictions of technocratic birth to reveal the naturally strong capable woman and her normal birth. (Midwives and midwifery clients use the term medicalized birth or even hospital birth to correspond more or less to Davis-Floyd's definition and evaluation of technocratic birth.)

More recently, the female body—once purported to be the universal basis for feminism—is undergoing a "destabilization." Judith Butler's formulation of gender is central to this process. Butler asserts that gender is "the repeated stylization of the body, a set of repeated acts within a highly rigid, regulatory frame that congeal over time to produce the appearance of substance, of a natural sort of being" (1990, 33). In other words, gender is an "act" that is intentional and performative, requiring the actor to reexperience a set of already established social meanings (140). Moreover, Butler notes that when the repetitive, regulatory practices that construct normative bodies are interrupted, opportunities and possibilities for rematerialization of those bodies–and their gendered identities—emerge (1993, 55).

If we accept that all cultural systems—not just biomedicine—naturalize power in the body in particular ways, then we must look beyond the impossible task of peeling away the "fictions" of science and biomedicine as if to reveal the true female body and the natural process of pregnancy and birth—or, as one midwifery client said, "pregnancy and birth as it was meant to be." In its place, however, a new task emerges: to understand the meaning and experience of natural birth in midwifery as an "effect" rather than some prediscursive reality. Dutch scholars Bernike Pasveer and Madeleine Akrich, studying midwifery in the Netherlands, for example, argue that women "learn to be affected" by and come to embody the assumptions inherent in their maternity care (2001, 236), be it midwifery or biomedical obstetrics. What has come to be known as natural birth, they conclude, "is not something that occurs all by itself" but is one possible "obstetrical trajectory" (Pasveer and Akrich 2001, 236). As one midwife in my study, Laura, put it, "even prenatally we have a culture for our babies: we have expectations."

If pregnancy and birth are gendered performances that are repeated within the "regulatory frames" of biomedical culture and institutions, then contemporary midwifery, I argue, seeks to reconceive, rather than retrieve, the natural facts of pregnancy and birth. Natural birth, as a critical alternative, contains its own discursive intentions: to promote women as potentially knowing, capable, and strong, their bodies perfectly designed to carry a fetus and to give birth successfully without the high-tech surveillance and interventions of physicians in a hospital setting. Further, natural birth is said to be empowering. For through it women may experience a sense of control and accomplishment that positively informs their sense of self as physical beings, as women and mothers, and also as persons.[2] In other words, midwifery in Ontario seeks to replace the predominant cultural version of pregnant and birthing bodies with what is in their view a better—but equally cultural—version by constructing and promoting critical alternatives to normatively (biomedically) regulated bodily performances.

Natural birth in midwifery at the turn of the twenty-first century, however, is not what it used to be. In fact, the apparently nostalgic ideal of natural birth is often clearly problematized by midwives and the women they attend. The construction, negotiation, and experience of natural birth in midwifery in Ontario both reflects and promotes a fundamental shift *away from* an essentialized understanding of female nature. Natural birth is being redefined by the political and pragmatic choices of birthing women and midwives in a clinical context at the interstices of mainstream and alternative health which emphasizes caring and wholism. New expectations of pregnancy and birth in midwifery in turn give rise to new gender performances—deeply personal, highly political rearticulations, subversions—that are *naturalized* in the body.

A Matter of Choice

Can the search for authentic or natural pregnancy and birth lead us to replace predominant cultural versions with improved ones? Ada is a midwife who comes from rural Ontario. Her training to become a midwife was characterized by a mixture of formal education and apprenticeship. She worked for many years as a childbirth educator and a doula before entering the Midwifery Education Program. At the time we spoke she had been practicing as a Registered Midwife for three years. After offering me an initial definition of natural birth as the opposite of medical birth, Ada began to hedge.

> Well, I guess the obvious thing that comes to mind is non-intervention in the sense of augmentation, drugs, episiotomies, procedures, vacuum extractions—those kinds of things. It's a hard one in terms of the medication issue because I would hate to say to a woman that she didn't have a natural birth because

she required some pain medication. That's a hard one. On the one hand, she did have spontaneous vaginal delivery, and pain medication can be, in some cases, very positive for women. I guess I shy away from identifying what clearly is natural; maybe that's what got us into this trouble in the first place is that feeling we have to have some model of what natural is and we have to have techniques to obtain that natural birth.

"So having a specific ideal of natural birth necessarily means that some women will fail to accomplish it?" I pondered aloud. "Yes," she replied. Indeed, a young woman in the prenatal classes that I attended said that she (herself a midwifery student at the time) would feel "ashamed" in front of her classmates and her instructors if she ended up in the hospital, especially if she had a C-section. Another woman I met several times at a midwifery clinic and interviewed at her home after the birth of her baby was apologetic about the fact that she "couldn't cope" and had "cried for an epidural" during labor and had asked to go to the hospital. "Next time it will be different" she told me several times. "Next time I will do it naturally." The inevitability that some women will fail in the goal to birth "naturally"—at home, without drugs, without interventions, without screaming in pain and feeling like they have lost control—is one reason that Ada, like many midwives, prefers to avoid defining natural birth.

It is clear, however, that more than shying away from defining natural birth, midwives are actively redefining it along new lines. Ada went on to discuss how midwifery care can provide the context for women to feel a sense of control even when interventions do occur.

By stressing that she's actively participating in a lot of the decisions; that there are still options—whether they are as simple as rolling from one side to the other. But [the important thing is] that she feels somehow empowered by exercising those limited options; that she has *some* choices, *some* decision making, and that those interventions occurred with her as the decision maker. I think the saddest situation is those who are left with the feeling of, "Oh, I should have done—if I had only tried the Jacuzzi longer. If I had only said 'no' to that epidural and tried another hour." It's those things that can haunt people. But if I really work with a woman so that we feel that each decision that was made—we tried alternatives and they clearly are [saying] "this is what I want right now." Then I think that women can accept responsibility for their own decisions. It is when they feel that they are pushed into things or even in the event that a woman has a caesarean—it happens lots of times in this practice—they are usually not bad experiences because of that aspect that she still controlled—not controlled—but she had input into the process.

Another midwife, Isobel, asserts that natural birth is a myth that says that, "if you are a together person you can squat in the corner and have your baby by candlelight (and) you have to have a vaginal birth to achieve some sort of womanhood." The myth of natural birth has served, however, to counter another myth: "that childbirth is so horrible that you need to be knocked out in the hospital." Isobel explains how her thinking about natural birth in the context of her work as a midwife developed.

I think that's really dangerous when you are making people try to fit into little boxes. But I started out thinking like that. My goal was to prevent caesareans. But I have seen so many women feel a sense of strength and dignity and satisfaction after a caesarean birth. And I think it's because they have given birth and they've worked really, really hard. Even like [when a woman has] an *abruptio placenta* and you have to have an immediate caesarean, it doesn't take way from it if you have that feeling that you are in control.[3] I hear this all the time. Women consistently say on our evaluation sheets or I hear directly, "I felt I was the one making the decisions. Even though I would have preferred not to have to make that decision, I made it, and I was ready for it, and it was great that you guys were there because I felt that I had a friend there, someone on my side to help me through that difficult time."

Making sure a woman has choices in labor usually includes a variety of things, such as where to labor, who to have with her, what to eat and drink, what position to labor in, how to manage pain (including taking pharmaceuticals), and whether or not to have augmentation of the labor. Very occasionally, ensuring women have choices in childbirth means planning for an epidural early in labor—not exactly the kind of planning usually associated with natural childbirth. This is perhaps an extremely open interpretation of natural birth, and even the midwives who agree that natural birth *might* include epidurals are quick to elaborate how such preferences are negotiated in a prenatal visit and during labor. Midwives don't want women making decisions based on fear of childbirth pain, peer pressure, or popular convention. Midwives explain to clients that if they do not have any pain medication, they are likely to have fewer interventions overall, feel better, and recover faster. They assure women that every woman can hope for a normal labor when everything's going well physiologically. Nevertheless, most midwives agree that when they have tried all the tricks in the book to relieve a woman's pain and exhaustion through physical and emotional support, an epidural can be "a blessed, wonderful thing." Other interventions too, as I have noted, have their place in the realm of "natural." Isobel concludes that "natural childbirth [is about] making sure the woman makes her own choices. That's my goal, not natural childbirth per se."

Gwen is a self-trained, urban-based midwife with nearly thirty years of experience, both outside the system and as a Registered Midwife since 1994. I got to know her and her practice quite well over the course of my fieldwork. She told me a story over lunch one day about a client she cared for named Abby who, after twenty hours of labor at home, was transferred to physician care and was delivered by caesarean section. Months later, Gwen bumped into this former client on the street. Abby introduced Gwen to her friend as "the midwife who delivered my baby." Gwen was taken aback at this introduction because she did not, in her estimation, or in any literal sense, deliver the woman's baby at all. (Midwives, in any case, say that they *catch* babies, not deliver them.)

In what sense, then, did Abby mean that Gwen had delivered her baby? Gwen described the labor and birth to me in more detail. It was a familiar sort of midwifery labor story. They were laboring at home, and things were unfolding very slowly. At each stage, Gwen explained to the woman and her partner about what was happening and what their options were. They tried different positions. They tried getting in the bath. Eventually Gwen, the laboring woman, and her partner arrived at the decision together to go to the hospital, and eventually to follow the advice of the obstetrician on call to have a C-section. It was not an emergency situation, and so there was a certain amount of time to talk about it beforehand. Gwen stayed with Abby in the hospital until she was brought into the operating room. Gwen and I wondered aloud together if it was not a profound sense of control in decision making throughout the labor—including the decision to have a caesarean—that allowed Abby to come to the remarkable understanding that Gwen had delivered her baby. Perhaps what Gwen had delivered was information and the space for the laboring woman to choose what was best for her and her baby.

The importance of informed choice in midwifery philosophy and practice cannot be overstated. As I discussed in Chapter 2, informed choice is an inherently politicized notion that is also at the center of the clinical practice of midwifery; it is intended to foster a sense self-knowledge and personal responsibility among clients, and create an egalitarian midwife-client relationship in which individualized, low-tech, even intuitive ways of knowing and doing are explored, valued, and acted upon. "The whole reason that midwifery arose in Ontario is because women wanted choice," one midwife asserts. Midwives believe strongly that all health care professionals, regardless of specialization, can and should take the time to explain the pros and cons of treatments and procedures to clients based on their clinical experience and the current research. Informed choice also makes room for more personalized information as well. Midwifery, perhaps paradoxically, then provides a rational framework incorporating emotional or intuitive knowledge.[4] It is worth noting that the ideological foundation of such cultural work lies in modernity itself, even though intuition is typically identified with tradition. Having choice is part of being a modern person and, as Paxson points out, making choices about sexuality and reproduction—from contraception to method of birth—is expected of the modern woman (2002, 216). Thus, the importance of having knowledge, having a sense of control, and having a choice during pregnancy and labor is fundamental to the definition and experience of natural birth in a fully modern sense.

How does informed choice work in practice? How do women in midwifery care understand and experience informed choice? Midwives explain informed choice as the act of conveying clinical knowledge to women and their partners in such a way that they can understand it and then make informed decisions about their own care. This may be something as simple as describing the importance of maternal nutrition on the developing fetus. Or it may involve citing the findings of a recent study on the effect of artificial rupture of membranes on fetal outcomes. Midwives also encourage, indeed they expect, women to read on their own and generate their own questions. They make this possible through their large lending libraries. They also stress that informed choice is about confirming and supporting women's own knowledge or gut feelings about their bodies and previous pregnancies in determining what is right for them. Midwife Isobel illustrates this in a discussion of choice versus risk, explaining that midwives try to honor women's choices, even when they may not fall within community standards of safe care, noting that this aspect of women's knowledge has been discounted in biomedicine:

> The more I see the more I realize this, that there are such gray areas, vast vast gray areas for what is safe and what is not safe in birth. Many hospitals would say that a woman carrying a breech baby should not deliver vaginally, that it's absolutely unsafe. And then there are others who say that she can deliver vaginally if it's a bum first not the legs. There is no absolute right or wrong answer really. A woman often knows what's right for her, and if she is scared and says "no" to having a breech baby—"no way"—well, maybe she *should* have a caesarean. Or if she says, "My body feels good. This feels okay. I can push out a little footling breech," then she's going to do it!

"How far will midwives go?" Interested in the dynamic between caregiver and client in such gray areas of informed choice, I press her to continue.

> You have to feel comfortable as a caregiver. I would say that I've told her the pros and cons. I've told her what the community medical standards are. I've told her the risks according to what we think we know. But if she wants to stay home and have her baby, I will support her and I will be there for her. You know she's taking that chance. It's debatable. Is there really a chance of a problem with someone who's always had a low hemoglobin but who's absolutely healthy? So maybe that's a normal hemoglobin for her.
>
> So it's the very end of line, and the woman says "I'm not going [to the hospital]." Well, then, I call the ambulance, and she is going to have to refuse it. I can't do that for her. So you call the ambulance, the ambulance comes, she refuses it, and you stay with her. You go that far with informed choice.

I knew of more than one case during my fieldwork in which a woman stuck by her plan to have a home birth despite clinical indications that put her outside the midwifery scope of practice. (In one case the woman had low hemoglobin and was advised repeatedly prenatally to plan to give birth in hospital. During labor at home, the midwife again advised her client of the risks and said she could not legally care for her. An ambulance was called, the woman refused it, the midwife stayed with the woman, and a healthy baby arrived without incident.)[5] Isobel admits that she has never had a situation that came to that because of the way in which trust between midwife and clients is built.

Trust, ironically, can play against truly informed choice. "How truly informed can informed choice be when someone really trusts you, and you develop a great relationship, and you put your biases on the table? You are influencing the woman. So, true informed choice is tough." But, she notes, trust in her as an expert makes women feel confident and that, in turn, helps them trust in their own bodies and what they can cope with or accomplish. Midwives, of course, do not offer informed choice on everything. Administering anti-hemorrhagic drugs for uterine bleeding after labor, for example, is not an informed-choice issue. Ada tells me this emphatically. "I wouldn't even ask her! If she was bleeding, I wouldn't ask her! It's not a choice. It's not a choice unless she wants to die . . . She's hired me to care for her. And that's my way of caring for her. And sometimes that means making decisions for her."

Midwifery and Medical Technology

Birth like most human accomplishments is, in many ways, a product of its technology. The artifacts of parturition, utilitarian and ritual objects, instruments, and equipment necessary for a culturally proper management of labour and delivery constitute a significant part of a society's birthing system . . . All of these objects, utilitarian or not, are part of a system-specific way of doing birth. As such, the magic they wreak is the same. (Jordan 1993, 80- 82).

The tools of birth in the context of mainstream biomedicine are thought of quite differently than the "artifacts of parturition" that a Maya *partera* might use in a cultural setting that conjures up romantic images of herbs and hand-carved birthing stools. Standard obstetric "artifacts" used in the management of pregnancy and birth, in contrast, consist of blood tests to confirm pregnancy and the routine monitoring of weight, blood pressure, hemoglobin, and glucose and protein levels in urine (which are indicators of medical conditions). Routine ultrasounds "confirm" gestational age and detect a range of visible fetal anomalies and, if desired, fetal sex.[6] Depending on a woman's age and medical history, she will be scheduled to have a range of further prenatal tests, including maternal serum screening (a blood test that measures the probability of some fetal anomalies) and amniocentesis (a procedure whereby a long needle is inserted through the uterine wall into the amniotic sac, and amniotic fluid is extracted and tested for the presence of an ever-increasing range of chromosomal

markers, anomalies, and hereditary diseases, the most common being Down Syndrome, Tay Sachs disease, and neural tube defects such
as Spina Bifida.) If a woman is overdue, "non-stress" tests to measure
fetal well-being and amniotic fluid levels will be also be performed,
and pharmaceutical induction of labor is increasingly likely. During
labor, medical interventions may include some or even all of the following: artificial rupture of the membranes of the amniotic sac, pharmaceutical augmentation to speed up labor, pain medication (including Demerol and epidurals), and continuous electro-fetal monitoring
(EFM). The moment of birth itself often involves episiotomy, vacuum
extraction of the fetus, forceps delivery, or a caesarean section. Most
healthy women with otherwise uncomplicated labors routinely receive
several of these interventions. "To obstetrics" notes Davis-Floyd, "society also assigned the formidable task of making childbirth—here-
tofore the primary symbol of culture's dependence on nature for its
perpetuation—support rather than threaten the emerging promise of
the technological model" (1988, 158).[7]

What is midwifery's relationship to medical technology now that
it is within the health care system? What should it be? While midwives are struggling to preserve the midwifery they knew before legislation, they now contend with an expanded scope of practice. They
use more technology to fulfill their professional obligations and to
respond to women's choices. These aspects of expansion of scope of
practice and increased accessibility to a wider clientele seem to pull
against the work of preserving midwifery and natural birth as a radical, low-tech alternative to technocratic birth.

One of the most basic understandings in midwifery is that technological interventions disrupt the normal or natural process of birth.
Moreover, common wisdom in midwifery is that one intervention
begets another. For example, if a woman has her labor artificially in-
duced or augmented with intravenous oxytocin—commonly referred
to by its trade name Pitocin or simply as a "Pit drip"—her contractions may come on so fast and strong that she is more likely to need
pain medication, which in turn, makes her less likely to be able to
push her baby out, which may result in prolonged second stage of
labor, which may cause fetal distress and the need for an emergency

C-section. A less extreme scenario is when a women has an epidural, followed by an episiotomy, and then delivers a healthy baby vaginally, but her recovery time is much longer than if she had neither. Evidence suggests that many of these interventions when used routinely are clinically unnecessary and do not change the health outcomes for either mother or baby; in some cases these interventions are the source of measurable harm to mother and infant (Davis-Floyd 1992; Hartmann et al. 2005; Sleep, Roberts, and Chalmers 1989; Thacker and Stroup 1999). The argument includes more subtle harms as well; women who receive pain medication recover more slowly, their babies are less alert and less likely to nurse right away. Some argue that the precious bonding between mother and newborn is disrupted by a medicated or surgical birth with effects that go beyond the moment. Midwives and women receiving midwifery care often state the belief that our tendency to rely on—or be subjected to—medical technology has destroyed our natural instincts about pregnancy and birth.

Midwives do use technology during prenatal care and delivery whether they are in hospital or at home. They use Dopplers–handheld ultrasound devices—to listen to fetal heartbeats. They order sonograms to confirm gestational age or check for certain suspected conditions. At home births, they carry oxygen for mother and baby, if necessary, as well as intramuscular oxytocin injections to stop uterine bleeding. At hospital births, they may administer fluids and some medications, such as antibiotics, intravenously as ordered by a physician. (They can also do this at home births in some instances). Some midwives are even seeking certification to manage laboring women with epidurals or to perform vacuum extractions (Kornelsen 2004, 5). Indeed, since legislation, midwives' encounters with medical technology are everyday occurrences. How the use of medical interventions and technology impinges upon the determination of whether or not a woman has had a natural birth is a subject that I explore further below. I also examine the role of women's decision making in whether to use medical technology during pregnancy and labor and how informed choice plays into the determination of what constitutes a natural birth. The first point to be made here, however, has more to do with the model of the body underlying decisions whether to use medical interventions. Specifically, how do midwives understand the pain of labor and how do they convey this understanding to birthing women? The tools of birth in midwifery care deemed necessary for the culturally proper management of labor and delivery must be seen in the context of how midwives view pregnant and birthing bodies as capable and competent.

Negotiations with Medical Technology

Giselle is a woman in her early thirties with two small children—the first born in a hospital in the care of an obstetrician and the second born at home in the care of midwives. After meeting and talking several times at the midwifery clinic, I went to meet Giselle at her home just after the birth of her second baby. She works as a graphic designer, and her husband is an architect. They live in a three-story Victorian house on a tree-lined residential street in a large city. Giselle told me that she "sort of knew" about midwives when she became pregnant with her first child but was quite happy with her physician at the time. Midwifery was neither legal nor publicly funded then. She sought out midwifery care for her second pregnancy because she was disappointed with the care she had received in the hospital with her first baby. She described being hooked up to a fetal monitor and recalled with frustration that everyone (including her husband) was focused on the monitor instead of her. She was unhappy with how her delivery was managed in other ways as well; she had delivered very quickly and sustained deep tears in her perineum. She felt her experience was typical of physician-attended hospital births and did not want to repeat it. When she became pregnant with her second baby, a good friend recommended midwifery. Giselle was very happy with her care throughout the pregnancy, delivery, and the postpartum period.

Giselle had maternal serum screening for both of her pregnancies.[8] When explaining her decision to have the prenatal test, she hinted to me that her midwife had discouraged her.

In the doctor's office [maternal serum] is routine, so I had it. But with my second baby I was extremely well informed, and I chose to have it. There was no need for me to have further tests because my maternal serum came out fine. Had anything come up I could have had more tests and determined whether the child was Down Syndrome or Spina Bifida, and we would have had to make a decision at that point. Thank God we never had to make that decision.

I asked her, "Did deciding whether or not to have the test give you any cause to worry?" She answered, "No. What it does is give you cause not to worry." While this is far from true for many women who have maternal serum screening—due to a significant percentage of false positives, and the nature of the test itself, which predicts only the probability that the fetus may be affected by Down Syndrome or Spina Bifida—Giselle contextualized her decision to use prenatal diagnostic technology in terms of the midwifery principle of informed choice. The difference, according to Giselle, from the routine use of such technology in mainstream obstetrical care, is that with midwifery care she was well informed and acted on the basis of what was right for her, rather than having the test as part of a routine at the doctor's office.

Giselle also elected to have one ultrasound because they weren't sure about her dates, a detail that could affect the maternal serum. Again, she explained that the ultrasound was both necessary *and* her choice. She was satisfied with the ultrasound because it "confirmed" her dates. (The baby, as it turned out, was born the day before the ultrasound dates.) She was disappointed, however, with the image of the fifteen-week-old fetus—"We could hardly see her"—in contrast to the image of her seventeen-week-old fetus during her first pregnancy. "It was just amazing. I knew where she was and what she was doing. I could see her opening and closing her mouth, and moving her hand. It was a beautiful picture." Even so, because there was no reason for another ultrasound and her midwives, she knew, didn't like to do tests without a reason, she did not seek another one at a later gestational date, deciding she would just wait until the baby was born to see her again.

Giselle's "informed choice" use of technology exemplifies how many pregnant and birthing women are interpreting midwifery philosophy and negotiating access to medical technology. We might not immediately recognize Giselle's behavior as an appreciation of midwifery's goals as a social movement to resist the medicalization of birth and the social control of women's bodies by patriarchal institutions. Her case seems to hold several contradictions. While it is clear that she prefers midwifery care generally, she is not beholden to it ideologically. Indeed, as we talked more, she revealed that she is made somewhat uncomfortable by the public perception of midwifery as a radical practice. While her family was generally supportive of her decision to have midwifery care and a home birth, many of her friends and co-workers were outwardly skeptical.

> I had one friend who was very opposed to home birth. And the comments I was getting at work were very strange: "It's not safe to deliver at home" and "You're jeopardizing your child's life." And other things like, "Do you shave your armpits and your legs?" It was a comment about midwifery care . . . There is a perception there that if you are going to a midwife, you are going to refuse medical treatment and only go to a naturopath, that you must be an extremist. But you don't have to be an extremist to go to a midwife. There is a good way of giving birth. There is no hard line between delivering safely and delivering comfortably. But some people feel that if you are going to go with a midwife that you must be an extremist and you must be trying to make a statement. But I just learned from my first delivery, and from friends' stories who had midwives, that this is not right. It's not that I'm bucking the medical profession, but in my case, I don't think the medical profession knows how to handle a normal, uncomplicated birth. They want to complicate it . . . some people just can't get the idea, that [midwifery is] not a statement. It is just the natural way to go.

Part of the problem for women making choices like Giselle's at this time is that midwifery care in Ontario is still a relatively uncommon choice and public knowledge about midwifery is still somewhat limited.[9] There is tremendous pressure to use medical technology because it has become so routinized in mainstream maternity care and the social consequences of not using it can be severe (Mitchell 1994; Overall 1987; Rapp 1990; Rothman 1996). Thus, paying attention to both the macro and micro contexts in which medical technologies are offered and used is part of understanding women's agency and participation in their midwifery care.

Giselle's understanding and use of midwifery might best be understood as an example of Margaret Lock and Patricia Kaufert's notion of pragmatism (1998), which offers an explanation for women's relationships to technology. Steering away from essentialist explanations that women are inherently opposed to technology by virtue of their closeness to nature or wholly oppressed by technology and the systems in which it is embedded, they focus on women's agency: what women do, rather than what is done to them. Women's responses and decisions around the use of medical routines and technologies, they argue, "are not simply those of either compliance or resistance" but might be better understood as strategies grounded in pragmatism (Lock 1998, 208). In other words, women use technology to achieve their own goals, but doing so does not necessarily mean that women accept the ideology behind it.

What do Giselle's negotiations with medical technology in the context of midwifery's low-technology ideal stance signal? Certainly, it is evidence of the persistent presence of medical technology in pregnancy and birth, with or without midwifery. That midwives now have structural access to health care funding and access to the socially acceptable institutional spaces and medical technology goes some way in explaining why their current clients may use more medical technology than their past clients. Prenatal diagnostic technology, in particular, was used fairly readily (though likely less than by women in physician care.) Most of the women in my study had one or more ultrasounds; many also chose to have maternal serum screening and amniocentesis. Technological interventions during labor were less common, however, among the women in my study, and were viewed with more suspicion than prenatal testing.

Midwifery's new location in the mainstream health care system, with access to public funds and medical technology, gives rise to a new set of negotiations with birthing women. Midwives find themselves increasingly engaged in the effort to preserve and promote a midwifery model that advocates such ideals as an egalitarian relationship between midwife and client, low-tech approaches, and home birth to a clientele that may not have previously considered these options. Overall, how women in midwifery care negotiate the use of technology suggests that women act pragmatically when confronted with imperatives of medical technology, on the one hand, and a midwifery philosophy that cautions against medical routines and technology they deem unnecessary, on the other. Clients like Giselle now make use of technology in a way that midwifery clients of the past seldom did—opting for maternal serum, yet planning a home birth, determined to avoid epidurals and fetal monitors. The notion of pragmatism adds a level of nuance to our understanding of midwifery, paying attention to its practice—in the sense Bourdieu (1977) elaborated—and to the subtleties of everyday usage, not just its ideological basis encapsulated in the notions of tradition, nature, home, and choice. Giselle negotiated the midwifery principal of informed choice on her own behalf, in order to have the prenatal tests she wanted.

Labor Pains and Women's Power

It's like, who invented epidurals? The person should be shot. Because, you know, if they didn't exist, people would just shut up and grin and bear it. There wouldn't be this anxiety. The worst part of childbirth is this anxiety of going, "I really want something. I really want something!" And then the guilt of really wanting something, because [you have] the knowledge of what it can do to you and your baby. And if there was nothing but the odd herb that would help you relax or something, then people would just do it. One of the reasons I had the baby at home is because I figured if I was in the hospital I would be getting everything they had! And that if I was at home I wouldn't have access to it. Also, I had heard a couple of stories of the guy coming in and doing his little pitch [for pain medication] on you while you are in labor—like a sales pitch! And I thought, "I'll crumble like this!" [She snaps her fingers.] By the time I was halfway into it, I remember joking, "can we get me an epidural by cab? . . . It's the same thing with these breathing classes. Oh, pain-free childbirth? It's not going to happen! You hear about the odd quick birth, the odd quick *painless* birth? Never, right? So if you knew it was going to hurt you'd just do it and shut up about it. If there was no option, you wouldn't say, "I can't take it anymore," because this is the only way you can do it! (Anna Lisa, mother of three children born at home with the care of midwives)

The vast majority of midwives recognize pain medication as having its place—if a woman has a pre-existing health condition that makes it advisable or if she experiences severe back labor, for example. But in the case of normal labor and delivery, midwives generally take the view that pain can and should be managed in non-pharmaceutical ways. The pain of labor is one of the main fears that women express in prenatal classes and appointments. Midwives do not pretend that labor is not painful, and they shy away from offering magic solutions, but they do offer clients another way to think about it and, in turn, to experience it. How midwives reconceive the pain of labor is key to their view of pregnant and birthing bodies as naturally capable and competent.

One woman in my study said that her midwives helped her prepare for labor and birth by teaching "almost another worldview . . . more of an attitude than anything else." In the midwifery model of pain, a number of things are emphasized. One, the pain of labor is not continuous like most other pain: Contractions are intermittent and build slowly in intensity, so one can learn to cope. Two, the pain of labor is "pain with a purpose": You are pushing out your baby. Three, midwives invoke the image of the universality of birth:

"Women have been doing this for centuries. Our bodies are designed to do it well."

Midwives insist that medicated birth is not usually necessary and that most women are capable of coping with the pain and giving birth with proper emotional and physical support. Midwives work hard to naturalize the pain of birth even from the first minutes that a woman goes into labor. They advise women not to fuss too much in the early stages; they should do what they normally do—eat breakfast, do the dishes, go for a walk. Likewise, they advise women's partners not to fuss too much about each contraction in early labor, so as to not give her the impression that she cannot cope. This kind of advice reflects an understanding that pregnancy is not an illness and labor and birth are not crises, but normal physiological events. Midwives sometimes talk about contractions as intense, not painful.

Leigh's story of pregnancy and birth with midwifery care is a good example of how midwifery works discursively to affect women's knowledge and experience of labor pain and how this becomes central (and desirable) to having a natural birth. When I met Leigh, a lawyer in her mid-thirties, she had just had her second baby with midwifery care. The first one occurred before midwifery was a recognized part of the formal health care system. It was a planned hospital delivery, with the shared care of a midwife and a physician. The second was a planned home birth several years later, with the same midwife as her primary care giver under the new regulated system. Leigh's experience of laboring without pain medication was a profoundly empowering one, her own individual accomplishment. She attributes this to midwifery's unique "worldview" of birth, which "has everything to do" with her confidence in her body during pregnancy and birth. For Leigh, midwifery offers a way to rethink pregnancy and birth, especially the pain of labor and the fear of complications.

> One of the things that I was so fed up with was this stuff about
> how people in our society put a great deal of effort in making
> birth scary . . . Most of the women I know are terrified of
> birth. Terrified of the pain. Terrified of the difficulty. Really

competent, interesting, smart women are terrified of birth. It is terrible that they look at birth that way; it is a difficult experience but it is also exhilarating . . . I felt really powerful after I had Martha. I felt really powerful after I had Zoe. I felt fantastic. I felt like it was my marathon. It was something that I had done, and I found it intensely interesting, too.

"Even in the moment? Even as you were laboring?" I asked her.

Yes, even in the moment. When you are in labor and you are trying to figure out how you can go with the labor, how you can help yourself dilate, how you can carry on through it, how you can let it happen—there is a long time in labor when you are dilating when you have to do all that work. And it's work that you can do. I mean your body helps you do it. And if you do it— at least for me—it is a very positive experience, and then at the end there is no more work because your body runs the show. But it's a very enriching experience because you end up thinking, "I did this! This was really hard and I did this!" And you can do it because your body will help you do it. You don't have to doubt that you can do it, if you believe that about yourself.

Leigh's sense of having a healthy pregnancy and feeling strong and confident also derives from accepting the limitations that come with pregnancy and "giving in" to labor: "The whole thing was a lesson to me. The pregnancy was a lesson to me, and the labor was a lesson to me. And it is a lesson in being almost someone not from our century." When asked to explain, she said that our medicalized, technologized view of the world leads us to believe incorrectly that we should over-ride the body in pregnancy and labor through tests and medications rather than "take the guidance of the body."

[My physician] had an almost antithetical approach, which is check, recheck, don't trust, trust means nothing, faith means nothing, gut feelings mean nothing. So that with Zoe, even when I was eight centimeters dilated and I was home all day and wasn't even at the hospital yet, my doctor phoned and asked if I wanted an epidural! And it was not a great insult. He was trying to be helpful because that's his orientation. But that, in a way, is defeating because it is very hard to be eight centimeters dilated, and I didn't even want the question asked. And that's why I was at home because I wanted to do that work without all that. And had I been in the hospital I probably would have taken an epidural at that point.

"Why was it so important to not take the epidural?" I inquired.

The reason I wouldn't want to take the epidural is because I want to do the work myself. I wanted to have that experience myself, and I feel much richer for that experience. And I feel like I've seen something that I haven't seen before, I feel like I've gained an insight into my body. And I feel richer for it.

The determination to give birth without pain medication was for Leigh, in her words, "a route to my power." She notes a clear difference between being in control of birth—something that she thinks is not totally possible on the physical level and something that midwives encourage women to give up—and being "in control of the circumstances of birth"—something that is possible to a great extent and something that Leigh and many other women cite as key to feelings of empowerment, strength, and even wisdom derived from midwifery care and birth. But does her birth without pain medication constitute a natural birth? Leigh says that while in labor she is "guided by something very primitive, but I'm not just a primitive woman." When Leigh describes the situation during her second birth—the planned home birth that ended up in a hospital—her ambivalence about the definition of natural birth surfaces and the line between nature and medical interventions becomes blurred. Because her first baby born in hospital had meconium staining, Leigh was aware of the possibility of this happening again and refers to it in her description of how she labored at home with her second baby.[10]

> After six hours I got [my midwife] to break the waters—partly because I had that meconium thing in my head and partly because I didn't want six more hours of labor. Frederick Leboyer would hate me because he said that birth is violence and that breaking the waters would make birth more violent. I was worried about the meconium, and I didn't really care about Frederick Leboyer. And also [my baby] was seven days overdue. So that makes the risks higher. So it didn't seem to me to be a bad thing to do . . . So I don't think that breaking the waters is terribly unnatural—people have been doing that for a really long time, you know? And if I feel like I want to break the waters because that labor is long and something else is niggling at me—which is what was going on—then I guess that's not unnatural.

Leigh's story illustrates the midwifery philosophy that birth is a route to the personal and collective empowerment of women. First, it involves the expectation that giving birth is hard but satisfying work that women are completely capable of performing. Birth is something that women do, rather than something that is done to them. Second, Leigh says that she felt a sense of control over her circumstances because she labored at home, away from doctors offering epidurals, telling her "don't try to be a hero, now." Yet her sense of control over her circumstances included asking her midwife to break her waters because she was exhausted and worried about meconium staining. (As it turns out, she was right.) She would argue, as I do here, that a flexible rather than fixed construction of natural birth strengthens rather than weakens its empowering potential because it involves women's gut feelings and choices—including asking for an intervention—in a clinically informed and supportive context.

Natural Interventions?

Kelly's story sheds more light on what constitutes natural birth in the setting of midwifery regulation and increased access to medical interventions. Kelly is in her early thirties living in a medium-sized city in Ontario. Her first child, Clara, was born at home under the care of midwives. I met Kelly at her spacious apartment on the third floor of a suburban low-rise building. She tells me that her interest in midwifery and her knowledge of "the way things should be" come from deep within her. She says that she has always known that birth was meant to be "totally natural and joyous, not frightening," and she grounds this faith in a kind of biological determinism. "As females—it seems very simple to me—we are born with these parts, with this purpose of our biology, and that's it. It's a process that happens, and it's supposed to happen. It's just biologically natural." It was through a course to become a doula that Kelly first met other women who shared her views about pregnancy and birth.

Using her own experience as an example of natural pregnancy and birth, she tells me that during pregnancy she did not take any medication or undergo any prenatal tests. She was getting information from her midwife about nutrition, herbs, and natural remedies. She was thrilled. "For example," she tells me, "I was having heartburn and asked, 'What can I take?' and she said, 'You can eat almonds!' " During labor, she avoided interventions too. For example, she explained that she did not have an episiotomy because

it is unnatural unless it's absolutely necessary. And there *are* a very small number of cases where that would be necessary. So, in that case, if everything else was dealt with without drugs or interventions—medical or technological types of interventions—then an episiotomy that is absolutely required would be—Now, for example, women who are dancers, their muscle tone and strength is so tight in that area of their body from dancing that they can't open up. Now they might need an episiotomy, and so if they went through the whole labor without any medicinal type things, then I would say that she had a natural birth, even if she had an episiotomy, because that was just part of her, of who she is, her physiology as a dancer. But it goes beyond the physical sphere of things. It includes your state of mind too. And if you stay at home to have your baby, you can add to the naturalness of it.

In Kelly's view, if an intervention is done because it is absolutely necessary, and not simply convenient or expedient, then the birth could still be considered natural. Moreover, she is suggesting that there are degrees of naturalness.

One evening at the prenatal classes I attended at a local midwifery practice, a discussion arose about tears that can occur in the labia and perineum when a woman is pushing her baby out. Ingrid, the midwife instructor, reported that scientific research had recently confirmed what midwives knew all along: that routine episiotomies were unnecessary and that most women did not require them. She then made a surprising comment: that most women tear during the pushing stage of labor. I suppose we were expecting to hear that most women do not tear during the pushing stage, a piece of information that would confirm the routine use of episiotomy as brutally unnatural. Her point was that most tears are small and either repair themselves or require just a few stitches. Even deep tears, in her opinion, are preferable to large episiotomies because the tissue tears only as far as it needs to and then heals more efficiently. One woman in the class asked her, "Are tears, then, a natural thing?" to which Ingrid responded, "I would have to say yes."

The room was quiet for a moment after that. The discussion then turned to what midwives do to prevent tears. It starts with perineal massage in the prenatal period, something that pregnant women and their partners do at home, to stretch the tissues that will have to stretch during birth. During the birth itself, midwives use hot compresses and apply pressure to the perineum to support it as the baby's head descends, crowns, and is born. They massage and stretch the tissues with olive oil to ease the baby's head out of the vagina. Midwives will often ask a woman to stop pushing altogether for a moment so that the baby does not come out too quickly. Giselle, for example, clearly remembers this part of giving birth.

> So with Georgia, when her head was pressing very hard against the perineum, [my midwife] stopped me, and she used olive oil. She massaged. And she gently worked her head out—slowly and gently stretching me. I remember the sensation—the widest part

of the baby's head had passed, and I didn't tear. I didn't tear at all! And they said, "That was beautiful!" It stretched so nicely, and there was no damage. It was just perfect.

Giselle contrasted her awe and appreciation of this esoteric midwifery skill to the experience of delivering her first baby in hospital with her family doctor. She described with anger how her perineum had torn badly when the baby came whooshing out to a chorus of nurses and her doctor chanting, "Push, push, push, push!" Giselle who was proud of having delivered her second child at home naturally, admits that interrupting the urge to push and massaging the perineum during birth are interventions. But she added, "If I was giving birth in the woods I guess I would have just pushed as hard as I could because natural instinct tells you 'Get that baby out!' So you would want to naturally push like crazy at one point." So, somewhat ironically, the intervention of her midwife in averting the instinct to push as hard as she could is what helped Giselle achieve her "perfect" natural birth.

Natural Intentions

The intention of the caregiver is another critical factor in determining the perceived naturalness of birth or at least the status of a particular intervention. The case of artificial rupture of the membranes is a good example of how intention and context matter. Although this intervention may be viewed as unnatural and recalled with anger or disappointment when experienced at the hands of a physician without being consulted first, women in the care of midwives do not ordinarily regard it as a problem. This is one example of the way in which midwifery is almost a gloss for what is natural, but this is not always the case. In a clinic visit during my fieldwork, a couple—Marielle and Tom—came in with their newborn baby for a postpartum visit with their midwife, Isobel. The rapport between them was warm and sincere; Isobel had been there for their first two babies' births and throughout the pregnancy of their third, but she did not attend the newborn's actual birth.

As they discussed the birth, Marielle began to cry, recalling how, long into the labor, the alternate midwife had told her she was not working hard enough. "I know she just said it to inspire me, but it hurt my feelings, and it wasn't true." Marielle was even more upset that this midwife had insisted on breaking her waters to "get things moving." She described how different this was from the births of her first and second babies, when her waters had burst naturally in the pushing stage. Marielle recalled how the excitement of those moments inspired her and renewed her flagging energy. She felt that the alternate midwife had not respected her natural birth process. She was suspicious of her intentions, and this played a role in her evaluation of the artificial rupture of the membranes as an unnatural intervention. Thus, the exception to the trusting relationship between midwife and client reinforces the centrality of caring and trust in midwifery care itself as integral to natural pregnancy and birth.

"It's more natural because it's more intimate"

I interviewed Claudine and her husband Paul together a few months after the birth of their second baby, which took place at home with midwifery care. They live in a modest suburban development in a small city in Ontario. They are both in their early thirties. Claudine is a physiotherapist, and Paul is a tradesman. In the course of our conversation, Claudine described both her births as natural. She specified what this meant to her: having options and making her own decisions in the context of a trusting relationship with her caregiver. Her husband concurred. In order to place their responses in the context of the broader life experiences from which they arise, I begin their story with how they came to choose a midwife and their reflections on the process as a whole.

Like many women, Claudine was influenced to use a midwife because a colleague she trusted and admired had used one. Prior to that time she had no idea that midwives even existed. Claudine and her husband were new to their town, without close family or friends nearby; the fact that midwives spend so much time with their clients was another important factor in her decision. Also, as a health care worker herself, Claudine wanted input into her care. As soon as

Claudine and her husband met the local midwife, Maya, and spent some time talking to her, they were convinced that midwifery was right for them. Claudine described their relationship with Maya as "almost like you had a friend . . . you could confide in her and that's what I wanted." But there was one hitch. Three months before the baby was due, Maya was informed that she would not have her hospital privileges in time. This was 1994, less than a year after midwifery was legislated, and many hospitals had yet to implement policies and procedures for granting privileges to midwives. Maya still had a thriving home birth practice, and so Claudine and Paul were left with the choice of either having the baby at home with her or transferring to a physician. Claudine had never considered a home birth, but they didn't want to leave the caregiver that they had grown to know and trust. They decided to have the baby at home, and everything went well. They didn't tell their families until afterwards. Three years later they had their second baby at home.

Reflecting on the birth of her first baby, Claudine told me she was disappointed with her performance.

> I thought I could handle birth with a lot more dignity than I did.
> But that's just me. I thought I could go through the contractions
> and keep my cool and, well, afterwards I was disappointed
> with that. I was embarrassed that I would be such a wimp . . .
> I wanted to be a strong person. You know that expression: Be
> a man about it. Take it like a man. The same idea. Just take the
> pain.

In fact, Claudine experienced back labor with her first baby, making labor even more painful.[11] In her husband's view she did really well—"a lot better than a man could do." Maya tried a variety of things to facilitate the labor and to ease Claudine's pain: suggesting different laboring positions, offering a homeopathic remedy called arnica, and getting into a warm bath, which Claudine credits with moving the baby down and bringing on the pushing stage. She remarked that most of these options, from the arnica to the hot bath, would be unavailable in the hospital. Mostly, Claudine recalled Maya just said positive things like, "You're doing great!" which really helped. Despite her ambivalence about how she coped with the pain, Claudine felt good about being in control and of having done a good job.

Paul added some details about the births of which Claudine herself was unaware.

> I noticed that Maya tried to keep—to stay back a bit. She tried to make it just between me and Claudine. And I think it's because you can feel freer with me [Claudine agrees]. And we had a relationship with Maya, but there is still that bridge area that isn't there, and she just sort of stays on the outskirts of that. Her main job is to actually—when the head is starting to crest, that's when she really gets involved [and before that] she's always taking her blood pressure and she sees how she's dilating and everything. I know now that she does that purposely. She kind of stays on the outskirts.

Claudine summarized:

> The way I look at it is that we can make more decisions and we have more options, rather than in the hospital having somebody telling us how it's going to be. And that to me is natural. I'm not one that's into natural foods and all this kind of stuff. I'm not like that. But that's how I look at natural. It's natural in the hospital too, but what it means to me is making my own decisions.

Claudine's view is consistent with the views of the midwives recounted above, probably for the reason that informed choice as a philosophy and practice is so important. But Claudine's answer also comes from her embodied experience as a birthing woman and the care she received from her midwife. It is all the more interesting that, unlike many other women in my study, she does not fear or categorically oppose biomedicine, and she does not fear the space of the hospital. She works in one, after all. Claudine had told me earlier that, even after having had two home births, she would consider having her next baby in the hospital. "Of course, I would want Maya there" she added.

> I mean, I'm sure they have good nurses there. And I would want to have some of my way too. And that would probably maybe make me look difficult. I wouldn't want to be lying on my back. But I'm not negative towards the hospital, especially because it happens to be my hospital, the one I work at. So I'm comfortable in the hospital, and I would be comfortable being a patient there . . . if something went wrong it wouldn't be the end of the world if I had to have the baby there.

A minute later her husband picked up the thread of what Claudine had been saying about natural birth being about making her own decisions.

> I like what she said. Either way it's natural because—well, I don't consider a C-section natural, but when I hear the word natural that's what comes into my mind: it's either a C-section or natural. But as far as the difference between them, it just seems so mechanical and production-line in the hospital. And it's less personal, and I think that we got to do it in our own house, and it was enjoyable getting ready for that. We got a closet ready with different shelves, and everything was there and everything was ready, and so, you know, it was just so much more relaxing and intimate, and I think that would be the more appropriate word— more intimate.

The interesting thing about Paul's answer is that he defines natural birth not only in terms of the body but also in intimate relation to other aspects of life—their home, the shelves in their closet readied with baby clothes, and, especially, his own awareness of participating in all these small actions and finding a great deal of personal meaning in them. In this flexible, social, and cultural realm of natural, he includes the intimacy between himself and Claudine, and also between them and the midwife: "It's natural because it's more intimate," he concluded, "more intimate between the father, the mother, the baby, and the midwives. We got to know Maya and I think that was very important. I don't believe that happens with physicians. I think it's very important."[12]

It is also important to point out some of the other ways in which Claudine was empowered by her decision to have midwifery care and her specific experiences with it. Overall, she aspired to give birth safely, with dignity, with input, and with support. Despite her ambivalent feelings about how she coped with the pain of labor, a clear sense of her power and ability to give birth well comes through in this narrative. For Claudine, natural birth with midwifery care is a matter of trust in her midwife and making her own decisions.

> Some of our neighbors said, "Wow, you're brave. You're crazy. You're insane." And people have never said that to me about anything I've ever done. So it does make you feel good that people might think of it as a brave thing to do. But I think of it as a way of trusting somebody enough—which is Maya—and having her involve me in all the decisions. Although she's the expert but it feels like you are involved in making them all.

Cultural Intervention

> How can our 'natural' bodies be reimagined—and relived—in ways that transform the relations of same and different, self and other, inner and outer, recognition and misrecognition into guiding maps for inappropriate/d others? (Haraway 1991, 4).

Do midwives and their clients perceive natural birth as the opposite of medical birth? Sometimes. "The idiom of nature sets limits," write sociologists Helene Michie and Naomi Cahn (2000, 55), in terms of defining acceptable ways to give birth. This can and does, in some instances, present a problem: women can be set up to fail at giving birth naturally. Further, it can go on to set limits in terms of gendered identity—as revealed in the curious but revealing choice of words Claudine used to judge herself for not coping better with labor pain, for not having "taken it like a man." Indeed, Kelly expressed similar judgment when she added the emotional state of mind of the birthing woman as a final qualifier to her definition of natural birth.

> I mean, sure you can have a natural birth and be screaming your head off through the whole thing—you know, swearing and cursing and that wouldn't be—well, it would be a natural physical birth but emotionally that wouldn't be a natural birth.

This troubling tension in the meaning of natural birth is often resolved by midwives and clients—though clearly not all, and not all in exactly the same way—by making the shift from a rigid oppositional meaning for natural birth to something more contextual, particularistic, and pragmatic. Given that midwifery philosophy stresses that every birth is different, individual meanings of what is natural are derived more from the perspective of birthing women themselves rather than from any rigid criteria. Midwives in Ontario and the women they attend are engaged in culturally productive strategies (both discursive and clinical) that move away from an otherwise taken-for-granted notion of natural birth. They see that it fixes too firmly nature against culture, nature against medical and technological interventions, and, sometimes, nature against women themselves (in the case of the failure to birth "naturally"). Such reworkings may also reflect a growing comfort with the omnipresence of technology in our midst and, quite literally, in our bodies. The new professional context of midwifery and the influx of a more mainstream clientele have no doubt been factors as well. Yet this cultural version of natural birth still works to challenge the powerful discourses of a narrowly construed science and medicine and the institutions of maternity care that have so far shaped women's embodied subjectivity. This cultural version is also profoundly modern, promoting the primacy of informed choice as a principle and an act, with emotional or intuitive knowledge validated in a rational way. Midwifery provides the context to say that choice and knowledge count, and women come to count on it.

Despite the clear acknowledgment from midwives that natural

birth is a slippery concept, it is still such a powerful concept that what midwives and their clients hope for and work for is often articulated in its terms. In many ways, the idea of natural birth stands for midwifery itself and for a particular set of gender expectations: that women's bodies are naturally competent; that with proper support women can handle the pain of labor and even find it empowering; and that women can trust their gut feelings in a context in which choice is paramount, interventions are negotiable, and trust characterizes the midwife-client relationship. In the language of Pasveer and Akrich, women "learn to be affected" by the gender expectations of the subversive idiom of natural birth in midwifery. In the end, we are reminded through these midwifery narratives from Ontario that natural birth has no static meaning and that it cannot ever be separated from culture and society. For indeed, as Marilyn Strathern has said, "Nature cannot survive without cultural intervention" (1992, 174).

CHAPTER FIVE

Birth Places and Midwifery Spaces

Birth Tours

THE HOUSE WAS UNDER renovation. Giselle—who is a graphic designer—and her architect husband, John, were doing it themselves in bits and pieces as they had the time and the money. The hardwood floors were rough and spotted with paint. The walls of the entrance way and the stairs leading up to the second floor had the look of having just been stripped of layers of aging wallpaper—raw but promising. Giselle told me how her midwife came "up these stairs, down this hall," followed by the back-up midwife and then John, arriving just before the baby. "The sun was coming in just like this on the morning that Georgia was born," she tells me at the top of the stairs. She stopped and touched the banister that ran along the length of the upstairs hall. She turned to me and said: "This is where I labored. Especially when the contractions were getting very intense, I was holding this banister with both hands—like this—and sort of rocking back and forth with my eyes closed." She demonstrated.

The room where she had given birth had a comfortable, lived-in look. On the low nightstand was a red phone that she used to call her husband when she awoke at 6 a.m. with contractions coming already five minutes apart. (He was in a sculling boat in the harbor, with a cell phone in a plastic bag between his feet.) There was the bed in the center of the room which she had leaned against and lay on. There was the rug on the floor where the midwives kneeled and leaned over her to take the baby's heartbeat when she was laboring on her side, near the end. And there was the place on the rug where she finally stood, half squatting, supported by her husband from behind, and pushed her baby out into the hands of her midwife who was kneeling on pillows around her feet.

For Giselle, the halls and banisters and bedside tables in her home were newly marked by the details of the birth event. The birth of her daughter at home had transformed the interior space of Giselle's house into a place rich with personal meaning and memory. Giselle was not the only woman in my study to give me a birth tour. Nearly all of the women I interviewed—especially those who gave birth at home—did the same. Lyn lead me to a tiny washroom in a one-bedroom apartment on the twenty-second floor of a suburban high-rise. Magali's tour took the form of a videotape that began in her studio apartment, carried on in the car to the hospital, and culminated in a hospital room, where she labored clutching the window ledge and gave birth sitting up in a hospital bed. Anna Lisa led me to a remarkable upstairs bedroom in a renovated schoolhouse perched high on a hill in rural Ontario; she had given birth in front of ceiling-to-floor windows that overlooked the sloping lawn down to the road. Lengths of sheer curtains blew in and out with the breeze, and anybody looking hard enough, she figured, would have seen it all.

The Spatial Politics of Midwifery

> With meaning making understood as a practice, how are spatial meanings established? Who has the power to make places of spaces? Who contests this? What is at stake? (Gupta and Ferguson 1992, 11).

When I began this study of midwifery in Ontario, it seemed that the spatial analysis of midwifery and home birth in North America had already been done. In Canada, home birth—unlike in many European nations where home birth has always been allowed—was a radical use of domestic space, the supreme example of women's control over reproduction (Rothman 1982; Van Wagner 1991); a potent symbol of an autonomous midwifery profession in Canada (Van Wagner 1991, 11–12); and a clear example of the trend toward the "demedicalization" of everyday life (Peterson 1983). Through historical processes specific to Canada involving the domination of physicians over other practitioners, the denigration of midwifery, and the rationalization of hospital birth in the name of safety, hospital birth had become the norm by the middle of the twentieth century. Home birth figured prominently in the development of community midwifery identity and clinical practice in Ontario as a social movement; it was central to their philosophy of care, it was central to their opposition to institutionalized care, and it was the primary space in which they practiced. Choice of birth place—including at home—within the new regulated midwifery model of care was a hard-won provision and remains an integral part of professional midwifery in Ontario. Further, the relationship between home spaces and embodied experience is central to midwifery notions of the body. Home is often posited as the ideal space for birth and the practice that preserves birth as a "natural" experience. As midwife Karina explains,

> I think if you don't have home birth, birth will become very medicalized. Home birth is the only way that we will know how women *can* birth. If you want to do an experiment about crops, you don't put them in a greenhouse. You go outside where the crops grow. If you want to know how women birth, you don't put them in a hospital—which is not a natural environment. That's no way to study birth. The only way you're going to know how women can birth is when they birth at home. Certainly, they are less nervous. They are relaxed.

Hospitals, in contrast, are not natural environments, according to Karina (and to many other midwives and midwifery clients), but they are now, nevertheless, midwifery spaces. The spatial politics of midwifery have become more complex, confounding easy answers about the meaning of birth locations and how these spaces may be gendered.

As midwifery continues to work to deinstitutionalize the location of birth and validate the practice of home birth, it does so now in institutional spaces through legitimate participation and authority in the public sphere as a health profession. It is not only the location of birth but also midwifery clinic spaces where prenatal and postnatal care takes place that must be produced or protected anew in the post-legislation era. This chapter describes and analyzes the new spatial politics of midwifery since regulation and public funding. Most midwives have moved their clinics out of their homes, and most midwives attend more than half of their clients in hospital.[1] My analytical focus on space as both a physical and discursive construct is another way of looking closely at midwifery as a cultural system and tracing its impact on particular and collective bodies.

To think about space is to think about power, even in, as Foucault put it, "the little tactics of the habitat." (1980b, 146). Anthropologists generally define *space* as the real or objectively verifiable things in space—houses, streets, cities, mountains, rivers, and so on. Anthropologists generally define *place* as the values and meanings attached to these physical locations, formations, built forms, or spaces—in other words, the realm of subjective, imagined, thinking about space. "A place comes explicitly into being," writes Berdoulay, "in the discourse of its inhabitants and the rhetoric it promotes" (1989, 135). The meanings of a place, observes Henrietta Moore, "are not inherent . . . but must be invoked through the activities of social actors" (1986, 8; cf. Bourdieu 1977). Midwives seem to use these words in the opposite way. For example, a birth might happen in the physical setting of a hospital—a place—but the *space* they create within that room can be an entirely different matter. In midwifery it is the space—the atmosphere or the "energy" in the room—that is discursively created, contested, protected. In the midwifery lexicon, space can transcend place. How, then, are places, including clinics, homes, and hospital rooms, produced as midwifery spaces and rendered meaningful? Who has the power to make spaces of birth places? "Who contests this? What is at stake?"

Midwifery spaces—including homes, clinics, and hospital rooms—are produced and rendered meaningful by midwives and birthing women in personal, imaginative ways, as well as by broader social, cultural, and political forces. Underpinning the importance of the relationship between embodiment and space is the midwifery model of natural birth examined in the last chapter. Midwives say that a woman must be able to "relax and let go" or "give in" to the process of birth. They say that one must be "in cooperation with one's body" during labor rather than trying to fight or control it. To facilitate and support birth as a "natural" event, midwives strive to produce spaces that are safe from the perceived threats of biomedicine and institutional control. These midwifery spaces are also empowering because they make time, room, and attitude for women to be capable bodies and persons at the center of decisions about their work of giving birth, their maternity care, and ultimately their motherhood. In theoretical terms we can say that midwifery reterritorializes clinics, homes, and hospital rooms, rejecting certain claims made about them and then re-owning them, making new claims about them and new realities within them (Ong 1995, 386). I begin with several descriptions and analyses of midwifery clinic spaces before moving on to birth spaces.

Clinic I

The scene in the waiting room at Jackie's midwifery clinic was always lively. Her practice was located in a medical building on a busy street in a large city. One of her most recent clients, Nicole, was standing in the center of the room telling everyone how long her labor had been: "Only seven hours! I thought I would know when I was in labor, but everything was so mild for a while that I doubted I was in labor. And then it came on so strong, I knew." Marta, another midwifery client, was sitting on the couch trying to quiet her baby by nursing. She looked up and said, "My labor was easy too—only two and a half hours!" She too wondered if she really was in labor until it came time to push. The discussion became more intense, and Nicole and Marta exchanged worries about breastfeeding—Nicole was having a lot of pain. The talk turned to tears and stitches. Marta had no tears and no stitches. Nicole had a small tear and a few stitches, and, as Jackie reminded her, "a baby with a very big head." As they chatted,

Alberto, Nicole's husband, changed baby Kiva's diaper on a blanket on the waiting room floor.

There was often laughter coming from the appointment rooms. Pam, the receptionist, was warm toward all the clients, their partners, and their children. She had a midwife for the birth of her own daughter the year that midwifery became legal and has aspirations of becoming a midwife herself. She spends part of her workday holding babies while new mothers run down the hall to the bathroom or midwives check their episiotomy sutures. Clients told me they liked the friendly environment of the clinic. Midwives often came out to the waiting room to greet clients personally with hugs. Like most midwifery clinic waiting rooms, Jackie's had bookshelves lining the walls. Most midwives and administrators draw attention to their lending libraries as important parts of their practice; women are encouraged to read to inform themselves on topics ranging from the clinical to the political. Among the most popular, most signed-out books in the practices I worked in were Eleanor Barrington's *Midwifery is Catching,* which describes the state of lay midwifery in Canada in the 1980s and profiles the life stories and practices of a number of individual midwives. Sheila Kitzinger's *Home Birth* and *The Midwife Challenge* exemplify the kind of popular, politicized, and clinically informative books available.

Videos and photo albums of home births are also available to look at: black and whites of a laboring woman draped over the edge of a bed, a pregnant belly mid-contraction, a woman's face contorted in concentration and pain, the crowning head of a baby close-up, the gloved hands of a midwife guiding the slippery shoulders of a baby out the birth canal, a dripping placenta held up for the camera, a baby at the breast, portraits of exhausted new mothers and fathers and friends. Anne, the other part-time receptionist, a long-time midwifery activist and consumer, commented to me that she doesn't like the "belly and crotch shots." She prefers the ones that show a woman's facial expression and other bodily gestures of the pain and hard work that are labor and delivery, rather than the images of birth "without a woman attached." The politics of reproduction, it would seem, permeate every corner of the room.

Bulletin boards in the reception and waiting areas overflow with birth announcements, thank-you cards, and telling portraits: a woman with newborn baby at the breast is flanked by her partner and a midwife, all smiling. It is a formal but intimate scene, like a posed family photo. Other bulletin boards advertise local services of interest to pregnant women and new parents—cloth diaper services, prenatal yoga classes, "funky, functional" nursing bras, subscriptions to *The Compleat Mother*. There are also articles cut out of magazines and newspapers on midwifery, pregnancy, birth, parenting, and child health, and printed notices requesting participants for research studies.

Jackie worked outside the system prior to legislation in both rural and urban areas and became registered in 1994. She is moving her practice to another town soon and looking for new place. There is an opportunity to move into a community health center (CHC), but she is reluctant because she wants a non-medical space. Midwifery waiting rooms are supposed to be for pregnant women, their partners, and their babies, she tells me. "They don't want to come into a place full of sick people." Jackie's concerns about spatial autonomy for her clients parallels concerns over the location of midwifery in the system. In one of the province's schemes to fund midwifery, each midwifery practice had to find a transfer payment agency (TPA) that would flow the funds to midwifery practices rather than funding midwifery practices directly.

At the annual general meeting of the Association of Ontario Midwives (AOM) in 1997, a midwife stood up during a panel on health care restructuring to state her opposition to funding midwifery through CHCs, especially if it meant they would be expected to share waiting rooms and clinic spaces as well. Should midwifery be forcibly integrated into CHCs, this midwife feared, what was seen to be for the greater good would be decided by men within the health care system who were privileged already; these men would decide what was best for midwifery and birthing women. She reminded the room full of people that gender is a part of midwifery's vulnerability as a group and as individuals, and she argued that for this reason maintaining group practices in spaces that are physically separate from other health care is essential. Many other midwives there that day also viewed this kind of funding arrangement as a symbolic and material threat to their autonomy. Some believe that the CHC approach is based on sexist assumptions that women should not be autonomous but should be working in groups, especially if such an arrangement is seen to prioritize the good of others over their own professional interests.

Clinic II

Midwife Laura describes how she and her practice group came to inhabit their clinic space. Leaving their home spaces was sad and difficult for a variety of reasons, not the least of which was that leaving home was a symbolic departure from the community midwifery they had known. After legislation and public funding, Laura made plans with two other midwives to set up their new practice in the neighborhood in which they all lived. While Laura was prepared to make the move to a medical office building, one of her colleagues insisted on renting a house, which was difficult, given zoning regulations. Eventually, they did end up in a renovated house in a commercial district.

> The choice came down to this: would we choose a medical building where it was all very clinical feeling, fluorescent lighting, no windows, being in a building with doctors, (but we would try to make it feel home-like) and it would be [wheelchair] accessible. Or would we choose a more home-like place like this and lose the accessibility? So we did choose this place, knowing that we couldn't adapt it. It's not accessible, and our compromise was to do home visits for disabled women. So we did a lot of talking about it, and it was our need to be in a space that was as home-like as possible and as less medical—so it didn't feel like we had joined the other side, so to speak. And that won out in the end.

"And how about your clients?" I asked her. Her answer revealed both practical and symbolic evaluations of the space.

We think it does make a difference to them that we are in this kind of space. We know that women are very comfortable here. We can have our prenatal classes here and we are able to have births here for those women who don't have a good home space. We've got a kitchen and a nice big bathroom on this floor with a huge tub and skylight. It's a lovely space, and that's important.

When she compares this to the home spaces of pre-legislation days, however, she reveals a deeper ambivalence shared by many midwives in this study.

Now, in terms of how people feel about the space as compared to our homes, I think the women who are new think, "Oh, this is so wonderful. What nice bright colors and there is furniture, not examining tables." These are the kind of things that we resisted getting into. But for women who had been with us before, it was a bit of a shock. For women who used to be in our homes, it did make a difference. One of my clients said, "Oh, my god. I hate being here. There is so much going on. It's not quiet and calm like it is at your house . . ."

I think it's important for women to know something about how we are as people. Know something about our lives. See the books on our shelves. What our houses look like. Who is in them. I think that it changes the dynamic between you and the woman you're taking care of. I am now a professional person in the office, and my life is not revealed so much. But I still talk a lot about my family. I talk about my birth experiences where appropriate. I talk about my experiences as a parent. I use them as illustrations of how I felt to be a new mother, how I felt to be working with a young baby. All those things are leveling things, and it's not just like I'm a professional. I think that those of us who worked that way in those days are much more likely to do that than those who come out of the [education] program and are given lectures on how to be professional midwives and that includes: don't be personal, don't become friends, don't reveal yourself. This is what it means to be professional.

Despite their best efforts, the new clinic space has implications for midwifery work. Laura tells me that she finds she talks less in the clinic's rooms than she did in her living room. The move away from home is also reflected in paperwork; Laura complains that there is no place on the client intake form to ask about things like the woman's family, her sister's births, her mother's births, and so on. This is the sort of thing she used to find out from women when they came to her home. Other midwives in my study who spoke of the contagious nature of institutional space expressed similar concerns. Raisa, a midwife who also worked out of her home prior to legislation, says:

> So, we have an office now with florescent lights. And sometimes you notice yourself changing a little by using the official antenatal records instead of your own.

Midwife and sociologist Mary Sharpe (1998) notes that the switch to office spaces meant increased access to technology—both clinical and communications—and to the network of health services and laboratories. Administrative support has also been necessary to handle the new bureaucratic demands. Working in office spaces now literally places midwives on the grid of the system—hooked up to new networks of communications, and the paper flow of bureaucracy, which they cannot opt out of. Secretaries, co-workers, landlords, couriers, oxygen tank suppliers, and so on come through the office on a daily basis. Being on the grid has its advantages too. Midwifery practices may be perceived as more legitimate, more professional, because of the buildings in which they set up their clinics.

The new openness of the clinic space, however, can interrupt midwives' work of being with women, of listening and connecting to them as individuals. Midwives try to insulate themselves and clients from their new location within the system by choosing or creating home-like office spaces. In the passages above, Laura and Raisa speak of the inextricable relationship between home as a physical space and home as a set of normative practices. By recreating home in the clinic space, home-like things can happen: midwives and women get to know each other, they can exchange personal stories, and midwives can meet their clients' families. Creating a home-like clinic space is also important to stave off the impersonalizing effects of being a professional. Nevertheless, a woman in the waiting room who is having her third child with midwives looks around the room and says that midwifery has changed. Though the rooms at the clinic are nice, she used to go to Laura's house and drink tea and sit in her rocking chair for hours. "Back then it was domestic. Now it's clinical."

One of the unique aspects of the new clinic space that Laura and her partners now work in is that women can choose to labor and deliver right there. This option brings the set of home birth practices to the clinic space and helps to confer new meaning upon it. When funding for a birth center in her city was cut by a change in the provincial government, Laura came up with the idea of having births in their clinic.[2] She got approval from their insurance company, from the College of Midwives, and from their midwifery clients. The response was overwhelmingly positive, even bearing in mind that it might mean clients overhearing a woman in labor while having regular prenatal appointments or while attending a prenatal class, or even witnessing a transfer to hospital, which is exactly what happened the very first time a birth took place at the clinic. Laura explains:

> The first birth that we had was with me and [one of my practice partners] Marguerite, and it was the end of the clinic day, and we were so excited and everyone was so excited. And then [the prenatal teacher] said that it was wonderful—she hardly needed to teach that night! The baby was born with the prenatal class going on. And also there was meconium, and we had to call an ambulance [for the baby], and the ambulance guys came in and out, and it was like a dramatic thing. And then afterwards we brought the placenta down to show the class . . . People thought it was wonderful.

Only half a dozen women have labored and delivered there over the past year, but Laura's practice is very proud to offer this option. It's a good option for women who do not want a hospital birth but do not feel comfortable in their own home spaces for a number of reasons—they may live with parents, have a very small apartment, or be worried about neighbors, roommates, or landlords overhearing. In one case, a client living out of town still wanted to be cared for by her previous midwife and so came in from a distance to have her baby at the clinic. The births that have taken place there are remembered as important events. They are part of the production of the clinic as a home-like space, as a safe and natural place to give birth. Births at the clinic confirm the flexibility of the space to be at once home and office, autonomous from yet connected to the larger health care system.

Making Midwifery Spaces

Despite the differences in geographical location and architectural style of these two clinics that I have just described, they are remarkably similar to each other (and to most midwifery clinics I visited over the course of my study) in terms of decor, ambience, and the way they are used every day by midwives, receptionists, and midwifery clients. Home-based and home-like midwifery clinics in the new system house the ambivalent intrusions of and intersections with the systems of communication, medical technology, and bureaucracy—the busy flow of professional rather than domestic space. Meanwhile midwives and their administrators mediate such intrusions, which threaten to make midwifery appear as if it has "joined the other side." Midwives try to buffer themselves and their clients from the new institutional context of professional midwifery.

Midwifery clinic spaces made of previously marked places of home and not-home are continuously and self-consciously produced, and they appear to destabilize the public-private split and with it a set of hierarchically ordered and gendered associations. These midwifery spaces work to challenge the knowledge, routines, and technologies of biomedicine by housing knowledge, routines, and practices that reveal a critical alternative: pregnancy and birth as normal, natural (as I have described in Chapter 4), and indeed domestic; midwives and women as persons, not just practitioners and bodies; and midwifery care as autonomous from but connected to the dominant health care system. Moreover, midwifery clinic spaces house gender expectations of birthing women as able to gain knowledge, as having a say in their treatment, and as physically strong and capable.

Theories of Home

> Certainly many of the struggles of Western feminism can be seen as a diverse array of challenges to the distinction between the public and the private and to the comparative value accorded to them (Blunt and Rose 1994, 3).

In the historical construction of space in Euro–North American culture, the public-private split can be seen as part of a larger multilayered cultural project.

> The private, *as an ideal type,* has traditionally been associated and conflated with the domestic, the embodied, the natural, the family, property, the 'shadowy interior of the household,' personal, life, intimacy, passion, sexuality, the good life, care, a haven, unwaged labour, reproduction and immanence. The public, *as an ideal type,* has traditionally been the domain of the disembodied, the abstract, the cultural, rationality, critical public discourse, citizenship, civil society, justice, the market place, waged labour, production, the polis, the state, action, militarism, heroism and transcendence (Duncan 1996, 128).

The private sphere was supposed to limit the influence of the state and to strengthen the family unit. "The home was considered as a microcosm of the political order with a male head of the household as ruler; women have been treated as private, and apolitical" (Duncan 1996, 128–29). Feminist critiques have long identified the public-private split as a problem. First, liberal feminism exhorted women to leave the home in order to participate in the public sphere by entering the work force (especially to take up traditionally male professions), choosing childlessness, engaging in "male" sports and activities, and traveling. Second, feminists sought to revalorize the domestic space and its gendered associations by opening up the private sphere to the gaze of scholars (staying home) and seeking to identify positive aspects about home. The assertion that "the personal is political" continues to challenge the characterization of the private or domestic domain as devoid of agency or politics.

The concept of "gendered space" emerged to take the theory of space beyond a crude distinction between the public and the private. Gendered space describes the patterns of men's and women's uses of space in both public and domestic settings, and the differential value attached to them by virtue of their gendered associations (Spain 1992). While the home may seem like a minor political resource and may not be ideal for all political struggles, notes bell hooks, it nevertheless can be an important site of resistance (for black Americans, for example, for whom public space is often hostile). While mindful of its potential for isolation and hierarchy, feminist scholars of many stripes have sought to reaffirm the home as a potential site of organizing, affirming social and political solidarity, and resistance. Anthropologist Lila Abu-Lughod (1990a), for example, describes how the Bedouin women she lived with and studied fiercely protect the system of spatial segregation based on sex that is supposedly "imposed" by the elder men in the community. For, in this space, she notes, women smoke, keep secrets, and cover for the absences of other women. Thus, the home should not always be construed as a space of oppressive containment for women; sometimes it is a site of relief or resistance. In sum, anthropological analyses and feminist retheorizations compel us not to abandon the home as a site of inquiry nor as a powerful political symbol. They remind us, in fact, that we could not do so even if we wanted to (hooks 1990; Martin and Mohanty 1986).

Anthropologists have not always been so sensitive to theorizing the home, even as they have amply described how social and political movements are commonly attached to places. Indeed, a proliferation of studies of nationalist, anticolonial, sovereignist, and self-determination movements show how ideas about nation and homeland empower such movements. Gupta and Ferguson (1992) further note that such place making need not be national in scale; notions of the countryside, for example, are used in local critiques of urbanization and industrialization. As key theorists in the study of space and place,

Gupta and Ferguson identify important new "sites" of anthropological inquiry that "take us beyond culture as spatially located phenomenon" (1992, 18), including the movement of refugees, migrant workers, and displaced peoples, the flow of mass media and public culture, and so on. Perhaps because of its location in the persistently spatialized hierarchy of public and private, the home is not as likely to be seen in terms of its "multiple grids," that is, in terms of its connection and contiguity with other spaces. Nor is the home always construed as a site of real political activity, despite thirty years of the personal-is-political kind of thinking and action among feminists.

Though the domestic space has been largely left out of theoretical advancements in the anthropology of space and place, work on the spatial politics of nationalism and transnationalism can nevertheless inform an interpretation of midwifery spaces in Ontario.[3] Joanne Sharpe points out that nationalistic processes share the same "genealogy" as Butler's formulation of the naturalization of gender through repetitive performance (1993, 98). Nations, she observes, are created through the repetition of symbols and so become naturalized. Smaller than the nation, territory, village, or town, so too are homes, clinics, and hospital spaces of midwifery naturalized as appropriate places for maternity care and for giving birth by the repetition of ideas, symbols, and actions of social actors, by the everyday performances of midwives and birthing women.

It is important to stress that in some ways midwifery and home birth were confined to the home prior to legislation. As with the issue of access to medical technology when needed, midwives need legitimate access to hospitals as well to fully do their jobs and for women to have their choices respected. Increasingly, social theory sees spatial boundaries as porous—allowing transgression, crossing back and forth—and space itself as hybrid, ambivalent, heterogeneous. The porous nature of boundaries between public and private spheres is exacerbated by new technology, mass communications, and new work patterns, which the example of midwifery in Ontario well illustrates. "Space is thus subject to various territorializing and deterritorializing processes" (Duncan 1996, 129). This is precisely what I am suggesting here, that midwives are disowning some of the claims made about home and hospital and then re-owning those places by making new claims about them and new realities within them (Ong 1995, 386). In the next several sections, I recount a number of birth stories that show how home in midwifery is imagined not as a site of oppression and containment for women but as the ideal place where women can labor and give birth naturally—in the sense described in Chapter 4. Furthermore, these midwifery spaces at home and hospital have implications for women's gender identities.

Birth Places, Birth Stories

It is trivial to raise the point that birth takes place *somewhere,* be it in the bush, in a hut in the jungle, or in a modern hospital. What is not quite so trivial is to consider that birth, by the mere fact that it is located somewhere, inevitably takes place on somebody's territory. (Jordan 1993, 67)

All birthing systems prescribe appropriate places for giving birth. These locations are determined by a set of interrelated social, cultural, medical, and economic factors and have consequences in terms of the kinds of resources and constraints present. Furthermore, the nature and spatial organization of the "birth territory" shapes interactions between birth participants (Jordan 1993, 67). Choice of birth place is one of the three main pillars of the Ontario midwifery model of care. In Ontario in the late 1990s, midwives were attending approximately 3 percent of all births in the province, with just under half of these at home. While the sheer number of home births is rising as the percentage of midwifery clients does, it is safe to say that in mainstream Canadian society the home is not considered the ideal place to give birth. A growing number of studies assert the safety of home birth for mother and infant, and yet mainstream medical and public opinion is often against it for a mix of ideological and professional reasons.[4]

Indeed, the prevailing public perception is that home birth is unsafe and that women who choose it are selfish. One midwifery client summed up the reactions of her friends and family.

They think I am moronic! Crazy! They can't believe that we are doing this! No one else we know has had a home birth, so we are quite alone in this decision.

Another couple told me,

You almost don't want to tell people because they will think you are a freak or you are irresponsible . . . So we really didn't tell people about the fact that it was happening at home. They would have just worried.

Midwives may suggest to couples that they simply not tell people that they are planning a home birth if they aren't going to get a positive response. Indeed, many of the home birthing couples I interviewed hid their plans from co-workers and even from close friends and family. One woman I interviewed told her three older children about the home birth plan, but they were sworn to secrecy when their grandparents visited. Another woman in my study went on a hospital tour with her sister who was also pregnant at the time rather than reveal her plan to give birth at home. Another woman told me tearfully of her grandmother's first words to her when she called to announce the safe and joyous arrival of her baby at home: "I still think you should have gone to the hospital!" We have seen how the hospital became naturalized as the sole location of birth in the twentieth century. How, then, are midwives, renaturalizing home as a place of birth? How is this struggle embodied by birthing women who choose midwifery care and by midwives as workers?

At Home with Labor and Birth

Jeanette: We did a birth once in a chicken coop.

MM: (raised eyebrows)

Jeanette: Hey, your choice of birth place: home, hospital, chicken coop! This couple was living in a renovated chicken coop, but it was very sparse. You know they had wood floors, and they were putting in windows.

MM: You don't mean a little thing up on stilts? You mean something more of a chicken barn?

Jeanette: It was not—oh, it might have been the size of this room. It had very low ceilings. They had put a little wood stove in it. It was the summer time. They had a futon bed in the one corner. But there were no screens on the windows. There was no electric lighting. There was no running water. And we do births at Mennonite and Amish homes where, you know, you may have a lantern to work by and wood heat and an outhouse.

MM: Do you have a kind of minimum requirement in that regard? Would you ever refuse to do a home birth?

Jeanette: Well, I guess if it was—safety would be the bottom line. And the thing is—I guess with our Mennonite and Amish clients—we carry cell phones but a lot of times in order to get called to go to the house somebody has to go by horse and buggy to a pay phone and call us. But that's their life style and that's their reality. And that's the choice that they're willing to make. And you know we talk about distances to hospital, distance to the phone, what happens if the baby comes before we get there. But you know safetywise, I haven't had an issue yet. We go in, and we do a home visit and make sure that it's ambulance accessible. We like to have a phone in the room where the woman's going to deliver. And can we get the room warm enough to make it safe for baby? So those are sort of like the bottom-line requirements. I haven't been in a house yet where I've felt like, "This is unsafe."

The "home" in home birth may call up images and stereotypes of an urban, middle-class, well-educated couple living in their own home or apartment. Indeed, many of the homes I visited for my study where women had labored and given birth fit this image. The walls are lined with bookshelves. There are gift baskets of Mamatoto nipple cream and baby bath wash from the Body Shop. There are piles of bright new Baby Gap clothes folded along with hand-me-downs. For the most part, these were the homes of young middle-class women, full of choice and aspirations. But, certainly, as the exchange above illustrates, not all of the homes I visited or heard described in the context of home birth fit this narrow profile.

The definition of what constitutes a good place to give birth is flexible. In Jeanette's practice, the midwives often see low-income, environmentally oriented couples or artists choosing to live as simply as possible. Many midwives in rural southwestern Ontario see Mennonite and Amish women as a substantial part of their practice. These clients' homes may have no electricity, no running water, no central heating, and no phone. Other midwives describe attending women in a variety of unusual places—outdoors on a deck, in a renovated barn, in an urban studio space with a shared bathroom down the hall—places that were either the only living space they had or places that had particular meaning and comfort for the women giving birth. As long as midwives can bring everything they need into a space and it is accessible by ambulance attendants with a stretcher, midwives will honor a woman's choice of birth place. In rural areas and especially in northern Ontario, midwives have distance rules, meaning that they will not do home births more than fifty kilometers or thirty minutes drive from the nearest hospital and its ambulance service.

Midwives stress that women don't need to have a perfect or spotless home in which to give birth; their normal space will usually do. Midwives don't refuse to do a home birth on the grounds of cleanliness or lack of facilities. As rural midwife Katherine explains,

> I've never declined a birth because of a dirty home . . . I think
> that if there is no harm to the family, then I can't actually decline
> a home birth because a woman has got a filthy floor . . . And that
> sort of stuff does bother me, but you know, it's outside trappings.
> As long as I really feel that this person can parent and has good
> support, then I have to let go of those sorts of things.

Most women give birth in their bedrooms, some in their living rooms, some in the bathroom or after having stepped out of a rented birthing pool. Women stand or squat or kneel. They lie back on beds supported by partners, sisters, or good friends, or sit on birthing stools. Large birthing balls (for women to lean or sit on during labor) and birthing bars (for women to hold themselves in an upright position during delivery) have entered into the practices of some midwives and can even be found in the birthing suites of some hospitals in the province. Anna Lisa was a fashion photographer living in a downtown studio apartment at the time of her first two pregnancies and gave birth hanging on to an antique coat rack with a futon draped over the bottom. By the time she was ready to give birth to her third baby, she was living in a spectacularly renovated schoolhouse in the country. There she gave birth hanging from a swinging bar suspended from the cathedral ceiling—her own birth trapeze—something her husband had originally rigged up for their children to play on.

Midwives make every effort to cater to the birthing woman's preferred position. Sometimes this means lying on the floor on her side with her hands in position to catch the baby as it comes out. Indeed, where the midwife puts her own body is an important aspect of the space of the birthing room. Midwives tell tales of standing for hours holding a woman from behind or lying on the floor at awkward angles to check a baby's heartbeat or a woman's cervical dilation. Some midwives carry scars and chronic injuries from years of attending birthing women this way. One midwife told me of having temporary hearing loss from holding her head close to a laboring woman's face as she cried out for several hours. Another spoke of a chronic shoulder injury from being accidentally, but forcefully, kicked by a woman in labor.

Midwives spend a lot of time talking with women about what will make their labor and birth space as safe and comfortable as possible. The most important thing about choice of birth place is that women feel safe. The right birth environment allows a woman to "let go" and relax in order to give birth naturally. The location of birth affects the speed and intensity of labor. A change of venue at any point can speed up, slow down, or halt entirely the labor process. When transferred to hospital from home, whether planned or unplanned, midwives observe that labor usually slows down or stops. For some women, however, getting to the hospital where they feel safe allows them to relax and let their labor proceed. Katherine told me about a woman who came into her care and was about to have her second baby at home. She had a somewhat elaborate birth plan that involved laboring in her own home and then moving to her mother's home in mid-labor to push the baby out.

> So I get called to this woman's birth, and I'm getting the routine about how we are going to labor at this house, and then we are going to run over to her mother's house. All right, whatever you say . . . So we arrived and we labored at the house, and finally we make the move to the next house, and when we walk in the door I say to myself, "I would really love to have a baby in this room too." The view overlooked all of [the] harbor and this huge willow tree, and the sun was coming up, and I thought, "This is why. It's the light. It's the feeling of the room." And she promptly turned that posterior baby as soon as she got into that room. And she got really moving with the rhythm [of her contractions]. So it was the room. There was something . . .

"That would turn a baby?" I ask.

> That would turn a baby! It worked for her. She had been working on that posterior baby, and as soon as she got over to that room she just went "Ahhhhhhh."

Katherine made a gesture with her hands, brushing downward from her torso to her legs.

> For some reason—either the light or the sound quality of the room—let her have a more relaxed pelvis, so that baby could make that little bit of a rotation. Or it made the contractions stronger so they could help with the rotation. She ended up having the baby standing up, which really shocked her.

Later in that same conversation, reflecting on the relationship between space and birth, Katherine observed:

It's the power of a woman's body and her environment to be able to work that kind of stuff out. So midwives take women's notions of where they want to give birth seriously. Including the strong desire to be in a hospital. Sometimes the power of going to a hospital is very effective; if a woman—particularly first-time moms and I think it's because it has a lot to do with the fear of the unknown. No matter how much talking you do about it, no one really can describe the pain. So once they are contracting, if they have a prolonged labor, they say flat out, "I can't do this. There is no way I can go on." So often moving into a hospital—that radical change in environment. Once you're there and you get settled into the bed or the chair, a woman can often get *cracking* in labor. So for her she may well have been afraid to let go at home because she didn't want to have her baby at home. She needed to be in the hospital, but she may never have reckoned with that, and as soon as you get her there, her cervix immediately starts opening.

The number of people at a birth is another key aspect to the space. One of the most influential physicians and childbirth educators in the natural childbirth movement, Michel Odent, believes that there should be no one at all in the room with a laboring woman (1984). For every extra person in the room, he believes, you add hours of labor. Midwives often mentioned Odent when the discussion of who to invite to the birth came up in clinic visits, prenatal classes, or in my individual interviews. Midwives accord with this view that, in general, women who invite a whole entourage of people to their births—"chanters, supporters, massagers, child watchers, and the people feeding them"—tend to have very long labors. Also, an individual person can negatively influence the birth space, especially if they are very anxious. Midwives say that they can feel it in the air when a woman starts to tense up or starts to "close down" in labor. Katherine, again, explains:

You can feel it in the air when a woman's labor isn't going forward anymore. And that is the part about midwifery that's the funky stuff—because you're sitting there, and you can feel it when the rhythm changes! It feels different in the air. It feels different the way she looks when she contracting, how she sounds. All of that is so related to progress, so it is important to always be listening, and if there are too many people around sometimes you can't hear what that woman is trying to tell you even if it is nonverbal. Because you have to really listen closely— it might just be the way she lets her breath out. But it could be significant.

One of the tasks of midwives is figuring out what to do to make the space right again for each individual woman. Midwives sometimes do "crowd control"—asking individuals to leave, especially if the laboring woman has requested it or is too embarrassed to ask herself. In this way midwives literally clear the space for women to relax, focus on labor, and let go.[5] The home birth story that I recount below touches on several of these interrelated issues of embodiment and space and allows me to highlight some theoretical insights on space and gender making in midwifery.

"This is my place"

I met Ellen at her house on the edge of a small town in southern Ontario. From the sliding glass doors of her kitchen, I could see nothing beyond the small stretch of backyard but hardwood bush sloping gradually towards a ravine. At the end of her street, there was nothing but fields and paddocks. She had seen the flyer about my study pinned to the bulletin board at her midwife's office the previous week and called me. She seemed eager to tell her story. At the time we spoke, Ellen was thirty-eight, working as a nurse, and the mother of two children. Her first one was born with physician care at the local hospital, and newborn Amelia—asleep in her lap—was born at home with midwifery care. We talked about both her pregnancies.

I do not like being pregnant. I hate it. But I keep talking to the child, saying "This isn't you, it's just that the distorted body image is a big deal for me." I had bulimia for many years, and so I'm still hooked up a little bit with that. So I don't know if I am just an exaggerated case—or if all women don't like the being out of control . . .

. . . So I tried to pretend I wasn't pregnant, and that helped me. And I did the MS bike ride when I was seven months pregnant, and that made me feel like, "Hey, I'm still a person. I can still do things!" Because you feel kind of—not really invalid, but more vulnerable because you can't run as fast and you can't move as fast, and you just feel like you are imprisoned in your body. I don't know . . . and I tried to wear clothes that I liked, not just big old frumpy clothes so that I didn't feel too far off the mark of who I was or who I thought I was. Clothes that hid my pregnancy. I just wanted to be unpregnant, unvulnerable.

When I asked her to reflect on her choice to give birth at home, she spoke first about what her home means to her.

This is the first house I have ever bonded with so readily, and it's also the first house I've ever bought brand new; it belies all the other realities that most people move up up up all the time and buy a bigger house and supposedly feel better and like it more. I have downsized here, and I love it more. Well, a lot of things have happened to me—just in my mind—about where I'm going, what I'm doing. Things have come together for me. So having a small house and having the baby here has really been so special. It was just I felt more at home here. I made some choices that were finally my own.

She elaborates on this sense of her home as a safe place, and as some-how significant to where she is in her life.

This is my place, and I'm allowed to be as I wish here. Every time the midwife came, she knew that she was a visitor here. She came to see the room a couple weeks before [the baby was born], and she looked around and she said "Well, that's a great chair for birthing and you could do this and you could do that." Most of the things that she pointed out were focused on me and what was going to happen to me. And that was so unusual and so nice, so special.

Midwives stress that an important part of the dynamic at a home birth is that they are guests in a woman's home. Ellen's in-laws arrived from Denmark five days after her due date but five days before she gave birth. Her labor started early in the morning, and she described to me the day.

I had talked to [my husband] Hendrick, and I said, "They can't be here when I labor. This is a small house and if I have to use the chair, or the stairs, and I have to come down"—I was fully intending to use the whole house to labor in . . . and Hendrick had agreed with me, and then he didn't have the strength to tell his parents to leave when I was in labor. So when I was in transition—which is the worst part just before the birth—I just said, "Get them out of here!" because I couldn't make a noise. And he leaned on the vanity in the bathroom and said, "Listen, Ellen, they've had kids too." And I just thought, "Get them out of here!" And then the midwife turned to him and said, "She would like them to go." So she was my *advocate* against my own *husband!* Well, Hendrick is a very considerate person and it really surprised me . . . because I would never expect him to say something like that, but obviously this was something that he had a lot of difficulty with.

On the insistence of the midwife, Ellen's husband asked his parents to leave the house.

Then when they left, my labor just went, and I had the baby. It was like it was some sort of hold-back because things weren't okay in my nest. And if that happened in this place where everything was under my control—what would it be like in the hospital? . . . So being in my home was so important for that . . . My midwife, she said to me—when I said "Hendrick's parents have to get out of here"—she said, "You don't have to be a perfect woman now—you're in labor." She said those words to me! And it just blew me away.

Midwifery may posit the home as a natural place for birth, but the space itself is not a given. Paradoxically, the home birth space must be actively produced. Ellen notes with pleasure the special way her midwife marked her home as a birthing place when she made a home visit a few weeks before the birth. The most obviously dramatic event, however, was when Ellen's midwife literally cleared the house during her labor by insisting that Hendrick ask his parents to leave. The words and actions of her midwife strike her profoundly, in part, because there was a contest underway for the meaning of Ellen's home at that very moment. The contest was only resolved when the midwife advocated on behalf of Ellen to say the house was a birthing space.

Equally important in the production of Ellen's home as a midwifery space was the moment when her midwife told her, "You don't have to be a perfect woman now—you're in labor." In Ellen's home birth space she was not expected to submit to a higher authority that always knows best nor to rules of good female conduct and civility if they were jeopardizing her labor and birth process. On the contrary, she was expected to express herself; she was allowed to lose control if she had to—no small feat, given Ellen's personal history with bulimia and her drive for privacy and self-control—while the midwife protected the birthing space.

Thus, home birth may be seen as part of the discursive intentions of midwifery more generally to interrupt and reconceive normatively (biomedically) regulated bodily performances through the promotion of critical alternatives in which women know themselves and have a say in a space that is both autonomous and protected. This story also illustrates home birth as potentially empowering; women can experience a sense of control (or carefully protected giving up of control) and accomplishment that positively informs their sense of self as women and as persons. Ellen's home birth has had a profound impact on her life, and telling me her story to me was part of it. As I left, she looked at me and said, "I will never forget you."

A Failure at Home

The potency of the ideal of a natural birth at home in midwifery is also illustrated in failures. Several of the women I met and interviewed had planned home births that ended up in hospital. At one of the midwifery clinics, I met Morna before the birth of her first baby. We chatted several times in the months leading up to her due date. We agreed to meet for a formal interview after her baby has born. Morna lives with her husband in a cozy second-floor apartment in a Victorian house in a residential area of a large city. In her mid-twenties, she is younger than many of the other women I interviewed. She had been working as a social worker before the baby arrived. Her husband, who is in his early thirties, is an ambulance driver.

As in most of my interviews, I started by asking her what she found so appealing about midwifery and about home birth in particular. She responded by telling me that she doesn't like hospitals because they remind her of illness and death. She described how two close relatives had passed away recently, and she didn't like the way they were treated by the hospital staff. In addition, she has done a lot of reading on the critiques of hospital birth, and "everyone" she talked to had had a "very bad birth experience" in the hospital.

> Stories like how they were only two centimeters dilated, and people were trying to give them epidurals, how they got multiple tears. And I just said forget it. I just know what I would have been like if I was in the hospital and a whole lot of people were touching me and probing me, and I would not have dealt with it very well.

Morna was well aware of the critiques of medically managed labor and birth in hospitals and was clearly concerned about maintaining control over what happened to her when she was in labor. Through the choice of a home birth, she could avoid the hospital and focus on birth as a normal, "non-medical" event. But she was also interested in experiencing birth in such a way that would allow her to feel strong as a person. Midwifery, she felt, offered her an opportunity to trust in herself and her body during birth. She wanted a home birth to continue to experience the sense of personal responsibility and appreciation she was developing for her health and the power of her own pregnant body.

The circumstances surrounding Morna's labor and delivery were unusual. She went into labor on a Friday night. Her midwife, Jackie, and the second attendant arrived in good time, and everything was going well. After several hours, however, Jackie was called to the hospital to attend another client who was having a planned hospital birth. The back-up midwife did not yet have privileges at the hospital where the other woman was giving birth, so Jackie was the only one who could legally go. When Jackie left, a third midwife, whom Morna had never met, arrived to see her through the delivery at home. Though she warmed to the new midwife very quickly, she became panicky.

As soon as my transition hit—that hour before you start feeling the pushing sensation—I didn't think I was going to be able to do it. I was like, "No. I can't do this. I don't want to do this. Forget it. [My baby is] just going to stay where she is." They kept saying, "Don't worry, you're going to do fine." And that's the point when we picked up and went to the hospital because I said "No way. I'm not doing this. I want an epidural!" I was crying and the whole bit. So we get to the hospital, and by that time it was too late anyway, so she came out naturally, no drugs, no nothing, which I'm really really happy about. And the midwives tried very very hard to talk me out of going to the hospital . . . but I think psychologically, I wanted to be where my midwife, Jackie, was. And I was really glad I did [go to the hospital] because, I had my midwife there, and I would rather have been at the hospital than at home without my midwife.

Morna's story reveals the instability of home as the ideal and always empowering place to give birth. For her, the hospital became the right place, the safest place, because the midwife she had come to know and trust was there. In the end, however, Morna said that having her baby in the hospital was her "fault" and that next time she would do better: she would do it at home. Midwives see the problems of having home birth set up as an ideal—loaded with expectations and associations and the status conferred upon women by midwives and other home birthing women (and partners). For Morna, a well-planned, successfully carried-out home birth was the mark of a physically fit and mentally strong woman, a gender identity she imagined would be played out and confirmed for her in the successful interplay between embodiment and space. Places to give birth, like all places, are tied to identities.

Morna's failed home birth story illustrates the potency of home birth as a political symbol for midwifery and as a source of identity for home birthing women. Her experience also demonstrates the relationship between embodiment and space which is part of the midwifery model of birth. When critics hold up failed home birth attempts as evidence to counter the claims of the safety and appropriateness of home birth and the cultural-clinical models of the body that support them, they rely on a false dichotomy between home and not-home to which midwives themselves do not necessarily adhere in their thinking about choice of birth place. To midwives, and to this anthropological observer, Morna's move to the hospital is evidence of the very link between embodiment and space which the midwifery model of the body espouses. When Morna moved to the hospital, she felt safe again because she was near her midwife whom she knew and trusted—that nearness was her safe space, not a physical place.

Often midwives find it difficult to mediate the strong desires of women to have their babies at home, precisely because of the feelings of failure that can arise if they end up in the hospital. Bridget discussed some of the feelings of failure that women might have who get transferred to hospital.

Lots of people who plan home births don't get to have them. It's only in a culture where home birth isn't the norm where that kind of [feeling of failure] exists. If a woman thinks she is doing something that is unusual or out of the norm, she is under pressure to prove that it's viable; she has to succeed at it. And if she doesn't succeed at it, then they will say that it probably wasn't a good idea in the first place. It discredits her choice and all the rest of it.

Bridget would say that the source of Morna's feelings of failure lies not with the midwifery ideal of having a home birth but with a society that believes that home birth is unsafe. Because home birth is not a "culturally approved way of doing things" and "a fringe thing," it is more open to criticism, whether you achieve that goal or not. Women may feel that it must be defended, and when it doesn't pan out, they blame themselves or, more subtly, each other.

Negotiating Hospital Spaces

Most midwives prefer home births. Some even say that when they attend a delivery in the hospital they don't feel like they are practicing midwifery. At the time of my study in the late 1990s, approximately 40 percent of all midwifery clients in the province chose home births. The percentage of home births, however, varies from region to region and from practice to practice. In rural practices, particularly those that serve Mennonite and Amish women, who tend to deliver at home, the rates of home births are higher—between 60 and 70 percent. In other parts of the province, in contrast, the rate of midwife-attended births that occurred in the hospital would have been around 75 percent.[6]

One might say reflexively that birth is a private matter, a private experience. But for much of the twentieth century in Canada, the only legally and socially sanctioned place to give birth has been the public institutional setting of the hospital. The experiences of women giving birth in teaching hospitals especially demonstrate the public nature of birth in the hospital setting. Midwives tell me that in the old days before legislation, before they had any authority in the hospital,

they had a number of ways of subverting the authority of the space—
by not following the institutional time lines and protocols. First, in
the case of a planned hospital birth, they would have women labor
at home for as long as possible before going to the hospital. It was
like stealing time from the public institutional space of the hospital,
and the interventionist management of birth. In addition, they tried
to keep women out of ambulances, if the transfer to the hospital
was not an emergency, by taking them in their own cars. Once at
the hospital there were other ways to subvert the institutional space.
For example, it is not uncommon for a woman to have a break between the transition and pushing stages of labor. In pre-legislation
days, if a woman was fully dilated but not feeling the urge to push,
midwives could suggest that she get into the shower in order to prevent the nurses and doctors from checking her and then "getting out
the forceps" if she didn't start pushing within minutes after that. In
these ways, midwives and birthing women managed their passage
from home to hospital, staying outside as long as possible and then re-
territorializing the hospital as a midwifery space in subtle ways from
moment to moment.

In the context of professional midwifery, as primary caregivers
with full hospital privileges, midwives still employ a number of strategies to maintain autonomy from the hospital for women as birthers
and for themselves as workers. They still like women to labor at home
as long as possible. They still prefer to drive women themselves if the
transfer to hospital is pre-planned and not an emergency. In general,
they also endeavor to make the hospital more home-like. One of the
simplest things midwives do is close the door to the labor and delivery room or birthing suite—depending on the facilities. This action
symbolically and physically keeps biomedicine out, thus re-marking
the hospital room as a midwifery space. Also, midwives usually don't
change into "hospital greens" when they attend a birth in hospital,
though they try to be appropriately dressed. As one midwife described
it to me, she simply brings her "tools of the trade" along with her to
the hospital.

These tools include her attitude—that birth is a normal process—
as well as her specialized skills. Midwives also bring some of their

own equipment typically used at home births, including a hand mirror (so women can see their own deliveries), a birthing stool, and a crockpot for heating compresses. Some midwives leave a cart of their own equipment tucked away in the birthing suites. Midwives encourage women to bring their own food, their own music, and other special objects from home; "anything that personalizes the space and makes them feel like claiming that space for their own for that time." For women who have had previous C-sections and are hoping to have a vaginal delivery, as well as for women who have had bad experiences previously, the hospital can be a frightening place. The midwifery scope of practice does not include VBACs at home, so midwives work particularly hard to make hospital rooms home-like for these women. Women are also encouraged to dress in their own clothes. As Katherine adamantly stated,

> I do not—absolutely do not—encourage women to use hospital gowns. I ask them to bring their own clothing with them . . .
> I mean sitting around with your ass hanging out of something just feels terrible! And then you have got to switch it around when the baby comes because there is no way to breastfeed the baby. They are the stupidest little gowns. And I don't like seeing women in them. It's like, now you look like you belong to the hospital. No. I want to see you in your funky t-shirt. It makes me feel more comfortable because it looks like her. There are the occasional women who say, "No way. I'm not getting blood on any of my stuff—I'm wearing one of theirs." And that's OK because then they are going to be comfortable. But most of us aren't [comfortable with hospital gowns].

Hospital births have implications for midwives as workers too. One of the biggest challenges for midwives as professionals is that they don't feel that the hospital is their territory. On the contrary, many midwives feel like visitors on nurses' and physicians' turf. Because they often spend long periods of time with laboring women, it is a problem if they have nowhere to sit or lie down. Nurses, meanwhile change shifts, and physicians may be called only when the birth is imminent. At home a woman and her partner can go through early labor together, just checking in with their midwife by phone. But if a woman has moved to the hospital, her midwife must be there too, even if the birth is hours away. At a woman's home, midwives can rest in another room checking in periodically until they are really needed. This allows the laboring woman and her partner some privacy as well. In the hospital, midwives may be able to use the physicians' lounge, and this has worked out favorably for some, but many midwives still report that there isn't a place within the hospital setting that they can really call their own. Despite legislation that includes them, midwives are sometimes out of place in the daily workings of the hospital.

The hospital is also thought to be a potential source of danger to birthing women, owing to the view that more interventions are likely to occur there. Many midwives believe that things are more likely to go wrong in the hospital. Women who give birth in the hospital are more likely to have fetal distress in labor and end up with a C-section than are women who plan home births. This is thought to be so even though women planning hospital births are at no greater clinical risk than the women planning home births or else midwives wouldn't be taking care of them. Some recent statistics on interventions rates for women experiencing clinically normal birth support what midwives generally observe: that planned hospital deliveries for low-risk women are associated with higher rates of intervention than are planned home births for low-risk women with professional midwifery care (Janssen et al. 2002; Johnson and Daviss 2005). "Every midwife you talk to will tell you that." Midwives will also tell you that one intervention begets another. Meanwhile, women who plan hospital births or ask to be transferred to hospital during labor are sometimes said to "know somehow" that the birth is not going to go quite right, or that either she or her baby will need emergency assistance. Several midwives related stories about healthy clients who had a sense that they needed to give birth in the hospital, despite previous happy home birth experiences or despite lack of clinical indicators to suggest a hospital birth was necessary. Midwives suggest that such decisions are based on some "inner knowledge" women have about where they need to be.

At Home with Hospital Birth

MM: What made you choose a hospital birth?

Richard: Laundry.

Nancy: We only know that now! As we were leaving the hospital, we thought, "Well, isn't this nice we are leaving all this bloody mess behind!" (They both laugh). But before— again, with all we had been through, I didn't want to take any chances. I felt that I would be more comfortable in the hospital, and we had enough people being skeptical about us using a midwife, if I said we were having a home birth—my mother would have freaked out! That wasn't my main reason, but with my age and this is my first pregnancy, I mean, its just—I didn't want to take too many chances.

Richard and Nancy had tried for a long time to get pregnant. They are a professional couple, both in their mid-thirties. He is a high school chemistry teacher, and she is a human resources manager for a large financial institution. Nancy's job is fairly demanding, with long hours, and partly because of this, she had been quite anxious about being pregnant. Yet, despite some tiredness in the first trimester, she enjoyed an "easy pregnancy." She found out about midwifery through a close friend who had had a very positive experience with midwifery care. Nancy did a lot of reading and felt very secure with her choice, despite the protestations of family and friends. Nancy and Richard were both skeptical of the belief, held by many of their friends, that an obstetrician provides the best care even for normal low-risk pregnancy and birth. They wanted to avoid an overmedicalized or intervention- ist approach to pregnancy and birth as much as possible, but they were concerned about the perception that midwifery is a "fringe thing," and they definitely do not think of themselves as "granola heads." They are both hoping that with time midwifery will become more mainstream.

When it came to think about where to labor and deliver, the choice was easy. They both felt that the hospital was the best place to give birth. Richard commented about their choice of the hospital.

If you look at the group of people who were at our prenatal class
. . . there was a big range. There were a lot of people in our
group who felt that they just had to have a home birth. They
had their hearts set on it, and I hope they all had them. We
weren't necessarily all the same, but the one thing that we all
had in common was that we wanted the birth to be as enjoyable
an experience as possible and to be recognized as a natural
process and to let it happen. I think that's the one feature that we
all had.

Nancy concurred.

I was a bit concerned too. There were people in our prenatal
class who were so adamant that they wanted a home birth. And
it's like, if you are so strongly in that mindset, then your birth
experience can be a bad one if you have to move to a hospital
. . . So I didn't want to go into it with, "I don't want to be in a
hospital or I don't want to have an epidural!" Because then if I
had one, would I feel bad? I ended up not needing it, but, never
say never! And [my midwife] Jackie understood that. Though I
am surprised at how acceptable it is that women—of course, they
will have an epidural. As soon as they are walking in the door,
they are offered one. People at work who told me that—it's just
astounding!

Nancy and Richard felt confident in their choice of the hospital
as the ideal place to give birth but also as a place where birth could be
"enjoyable" and "natural" as possible. Nancy was comfortable with
the possibility that she might need or want an epidural or other interventions only available in hospital. But she was also wary of what
she knew of standard hospital procedures with regard to pain management, and she wanted to protect herself against the possibility of being
pressured to have an epidural the minute she walked in the door. Her
midwife supported her choice of birth place and suggested ways to
personalize the hospital space and to make it home-like by bringing
their own food and their own clothes.

Their daughter was born three weeks before her due date. Nancy awoke at three o'clock in the morning with what she thought was false labor; menstrual-like cramps coming every ten minutes. She was supposed to be at the office that morning and debated going in. They tried to "walk it off," but she had a few contractions on the way to the supermarket. So they bought the dried fruit and Gatorade they had planned to take to the hospital—"enough for both of us and enough for a long, long labor," Nancy recalled. By the time they got home, the contractions had not subsided, and only then did they realize that Nancy was really in labor. About eleven o'clock Nancy sent Richard to clean the bathroom so she could sit in the bath to labor and so that it would be clean for guests coming to see the baby afterwards. Richard cleaned the bathroom while Nancy timed her contractions.

By noon the contractions were coming regularly. They called Jackie, their midwife, and arranged to meet her at the hospital. They went straight to the labor and delivery unit, and by then Nancy's contractions were quite painful. Jackie arrived and immediately checked her cervical dilation.

> I was already eight or nine centimeters! Richard said, "Holy shit!" And I said, "Oh, you mean I really am in labor? Like, did I miss a prenatal class or something?" So when I arrived I was eight or nine centimeters, and it really hadn't been that bad. Maybe the last hour or so had been but . . . and then we started to push at around two o'clock and [the baby] came at three o'clock. So it was all very easy, and it didn't last very long, and it wasn't all that painful. I haven't even described it as being painful. It wasn't pain. It was more like discomfort, even the most painful part of it. We had a really good experience.

Throughout the labor and delivery, Jackie encouraged visualization and vocalization. As Nancy recalled,

> I would vocalize "open open open." I would say the words. And Jackie encouraged that. It was like a moan. And my visualization—our shower curtain is a field of purple irises

and that's what I kept thinking about was that image of them opening . . . I think that it made me manage the pain better. It gave me something to think about. I'm a very visual person and I like purple, and it gave me something to focus on, to think about that opening instead of what was going on in my body, because my body was sort of on its own and my mind was sort of saying, "Well, what am I supposed to do?"

Jackie kept saying, "You have to push through the pain," and it suddenly dawned on me that these people who were around me weren't going to let me leave until I had pushed through the pain. And with that I really pushed, and that's when [my baby] popped out.

Jackie had described to me how she liked to help women think about their bodies in labor and birth.[7] During the pushing stage of labor, midwives tell women over and over, "You are stretching beautifully," referring to the intense stretching of the perineum as the baby's head crowns. Specifically, Jackie encourages women not to try to control each contraction nor to be out of control but rather to be "in cooperation with your body." Nancy reminded herself of this during labor when things were getting more intense and difficult, and she tried to work with her body instead of against it. Jackie observes that conveying this notion of being in cooperation with your body really works for women. As Nancy said, "Once I really understood what that was, my labor became much easier." "Were there any interventions at all used in the hospital?" I asked. "No," was the reply, "except for olive oil and hot compresses applied to the perineum during the pushing stage." These particular "interventions" were familiar to me from home birth stories and from the home births that I attended as part of my research. Using the space of the hospital in the same way they would use a home birth space, Nancy's midwives naturalized the hospital as a good place to give birth. Midwives and birthing women make the place their own.

Other women in my study had chosen hospital births for similar reasons. Magali, a Polish/French Canadian woman chose a hospital birth for her second baby, despite what she describes as a terrible and humiliating experience in a teaching hospital with her first baby. "Here at home your neighbors can hear you scream," she told me. "And I don't like that. Also, it's a mess afterwards. You have to clean." Thus, her concern for privacy and care, which included cleaning, was addressed by having a hospital birth, but this time with midwifery care. For Magali, it was midwifery care itself that made her second birth "more natural" (even though the first time she didn't have pain medications or interventions). The location of her birth was less important. "I see midwifery as something about humanity," she told me. "We have to be treated well, you know? And birth should be good experience. It should be well done." In a further twist, she brought a video camera and a tripod along to the hospital and videotaped the entire event. Not only was she comfortable laboring and giving birth in front of the camera, but she called out to her husband and her midwives several times between contractions to check the angle of the camera, so it wouldn't miss anything. We watched the videotape together on one of my visits to her apartment, but she was not in the habit of showing it to others. She intended to show it to her son when he grew up.

As part of my regular set of interview questions, I asked women if midwifery care taught them anything about their bodies. Almost invariably, they spoke, as Nancy did, of a sense of a new confidence in their bodies to be pregnant and to give birth well. Midwives told me again and again that one of the goals of their work was realized when a woman could look up after pushing her baby out and say, "I did it!" instead of "Thank you for delivering my baby." Nancy's own reflections of her embodied experience with birth attended by a midwife in the hospital bear this out.

> I didn't think that I could do it before . . . Jackie was very much, "You can do this!" all the way through. Of course you can do this, and here's how you are going to do it. And we are here to help you and support you and yes you can do it. Your body says you can do it. Your mind is the one that has to be convinced.

If both mother and baby are well, postpartum care, regardless of where the birth takes place, is conducted in the home. Midwives often leave the hospital with the woman only a few hours after birth or meet her at her home the next day if she stays overnight. Postpartum visits at home may take place once every few days or even every day after a birth for about a week, depending on the particular needs of the new mother and baby. Like most midwifery clients, Richard and Nancy raved about it.

> The post partum really made the difference. I knew that Jackie was going to be there every day and that I could ask any question, and she was there. And I can't imagine—I mean I'm thirty-five years old. I've read all the books. I've got lots of friends that I can call on. I've got my sister. But even so I needed to have that one-on-one for breastfeeding and for taking care of me, too. I mean, it was like, "Let's look at my nipples. Are they OK?" You know, this frank discussion! I can't imagine having—I don't have confidence that a doctor could really say whether or not my nipples were OK, you know?

Nancy and Richard, and Magali and her husband are at home, so to speak, with hospital birth. It feels safe to them. It feels natural. Nancy's birth story, while perhaps unusual in that she describes it as relatively easy, is otherwise typical of women's experience giving birth under the care of midwives at home or in the hospital. Magali is less concerned with the physical location of birth as with the privacy and dignity she found with midwifery care. Though they were all concerned with past and potential interference they associated with the hospital—such as epidurals and teaching rounds—midwifery care mediates the space for them in important ways, mitigating against the institutional feel and its potential embodied effects.

Midwifery Spaces and Expectations

> Space that has been seized upon by the imagination cannot remain indifferent space subject to measures and estimates of the

survey. It has been lived in, not in its positivity, but with all the partiality of imagination (Bachelard 1958, xxxii).

Home, as the ideal space for childbirth, remains a symbol for the new midwifery in Ontario and for natural birth as it transitions from outside in the community to (sometimes) inside the health care system. Perhaps the fundamental project of midwifery no longer appears so radical—to follow women's pregnancies and births with continuous care, to inform them of their clinical options at all times, to authorize their own choices, and to allow them the choice of birth place. However, we are reminded in these stories that home and home-like clinic and hospital spaces are not given but must be made out of places with already conventional meanings and uses. Sometimes these midwifery spaces exist only temporarily; often they must compete with other uses and meanings. In the pursuit of home as the ideal place for natural pregnancy and birth, midwives and the women they care for reterritorialize clinics, homes, and hospital rooms in personal, imaginative ways, as well as in ways that speak to the political context of midwifery in Ontario. This context includes clinical debates about the safety and appropriateness of home birth (which themselves are bound up in ideological and professional concerns of physicians and hospitals), as well as issues surrounding the funding of midwifery services, the physical locations of clinics, and the autonomy of midwives as professionals.

Making midwifery spaces at home or in the hospital challenges biomedical knowledge, routines, and technologies, creating a counterdiscourse with its own rhetoric and tactics that facilitates the practice and performance of the mind-body unity. As midwifery spaces are imagined, known, lived in, struggled over, and remembered, so are particular gender expectations of women as knowing subjects and capable bodies in the important processes of pregnancy, labor, and birth fostered. Further, the conspicuously modern values of flexibility and choice are ensconced in contemporary midwifery's cultural project—in its cultural negotiation of gender—offering a critical alternative with the potential to transform gender expectations and naturalize them in the body.

The Politics of
Representation Revisited

O N THE EVE OF completing this book, I received an e-mail
from a self-described "home birth midwife in rural Pennsyl-
vania," who wrote that she had been recently introduced to
my work by an American obstetrician known as Dr Amy. Dr Amy,
I soon discovered, is an obstetrician-gynecologist who hosts an in-
formational web site about pregnancy and childbirth called "Ask Dr
Amy" and writes a number of topically related blogs, including "The
home birth debate." "She is using excerpts from your work" the midwife wrote, "to prove her biased points [against home birth and natural birth] and I fear it misrepresents you." She directed me to the web
link so I could see for myself. On Thursday, June 15, 2006, Dr Amy
had written, "There is a fascinating article in this month's *Medical
Anthropology Quarterly* about midwifery in Canada and the definition
of 'natural' birth. This article confirms my assertion that 'normal' or
'natural' birth is merely a social construction." Her post continues at
length, quoting my article directly. The next day she posted a second
blog entry concerning my article entitled "The Troubling Moral Implications of 'Natural' Birth." My article, she argued, proved that

> "natural" birth is used as a cudgel for some women . . . to beat
> other women over the head. It is an arbitrary definition that
> includes what advocates want and excludes what they don't want.
> They have every right to adopt social and cultural constructs

about birth that they wish to adopt. However, it is important for everyone to understand that their views are arbitrary and tell us nothing about what type of birth is better than any other.

I was intrigued and appalled, but perhaps I should not have been surprised. Indeed, it was precisely what I feared could happen when my work was published. I responded the following day with this post:

Perhaps the first thing to be said is that anthropologists tend to view physiological processes like birth as culturally shaped by their participants. So when I state that natural birth is a cultural construction, I do not mean it is "merely" arbitrary or made up as if in contrast to some biomedical reality . . . In other words, midwives are seeking to actively shape pregnancy and birth into what they consider a better cultural model for birth in a society where the predominant cultural model for birth has been amply demonstrated as sending fairly negative messages about women's "nature." Perhaps not all midwives across North America see their work this way, but this is what I saw happening in Ontario in the late 1990s.

I also want to stress that to critically analyse a concept or practice, as I have done in the case of natural birth in midwifery, is not to dismiss or expose it as false or artificial. And while I do agree with Dr Amy that the ideal of natural birth can work against women, what I found most interesting, as an anthropologist, was how midwives themselves were critically aware of this and thus were reflecting on their own work, their own ideals. However, my critique of natural birth in this article should not be misconstrued as some sort of exposé of midwifery's manipulative use of a false ideal, but rather an exploration of a dynamic cultural system co-created by midwives and the women they care for.

By this point, many other commentators—mostly detractors of Dr Amy's views—had waded into the debate. The tone of the on-line discussion ranged from thoughtful to frustrated to hostile. Dr Amy responded to the general readership of the blog:

> If "natural" childbirth includes all sorts of unnatural things like blood pressure monitoring and waterbirth, then the adjective "natural" is inappropriate on its face . . . Advocates can call their preferences Bradley birth, Lamaze, etc., etc., but they are not entitled to call their personal preferences "natural childbirth" . . . I don't know how to make it any clearer than I have made it. Natural childbirth no longer exists.

I had to agree with her final pronouncement—sort of—to the extent that my purpose in this book has been to describe how the midwifery ideal of nature is being redefined and relived. My approach has been Foucauldian in that I do not take a stand on the existence of such supposedly natural categories as human nature but rather pursue the question of how such concepts are played out in social, political, and lived bodies (cf. Rabinow 1994). The problem is that while Dr Amy, by using my research in the service of her own agenda, was comfortable arguing that "midwives are constructing a cultural model, not revealing a hitherto unappreciated scientific truth," she was less keen to say the same for mainstream obstetric medicine.

The day after my first post, she graciously thanked me on the blog for taking the time to participate in the debate. She also had a further question for me: "Are different culturally derived understandings of childbirth equal, or does one culture have the right to claim superiority?" I replied,

> Traditional obstetric methods are not superior in every way when it comes childbirth, as scientific evidence is now demonstrating. The superiority complex of obstetric medicine has damaged other cultural birthing systems unnecessarily. For example, anthropologists have documented the loss of many effective birthing techniques—such as upright birth—when medical missionaries to the colonies tried to stamp it out and retrain local midwives in the biomedical custom of the lithotomy position.

The lithotomy position was considered superior not because it was proven to make childbirth safer or easier for mother and baby but rather because it was thought to be "more civilized." So the assumption of "superiority" is a dangerous platform on which to deride or suppress other birthing systems. That said, there are many demonstrably life saving techniques and medicines that should be made available when necessary. Anthropologists studying childbirth generally advocate what has been coined "mutual accommodation" between systems.

Also it must be said that obstetrics, as the dominant system in Europe and North America, takes its superiority for granted, and has been allowed to do so not always on the basis of clinical superiority, but because of the social and economic power it wields, and the faith we as a society tend to put in science and medicine.

I have recounted this incident because it illustrates some important things about the nature of debates around midwifery, natural birth, and home birth. First, the use of my academic work on a public blog speaks directly to the politics of representation. In the introduction, I stated that one of my public intellectual goals in this work was to bring new stories to light to serve as counterpoints to hegemonic biomedical stories about pregnancy, birth, and birth attendance. At the same time, I stated that I was concerned about the potential social and political consequences of making midwifery more visible for midwives and women who participated in my study at what is still a vulnerable time. However, I think now that the existence of the blog—and the appearance of my work on it—is simply further evidence that the transformation of midwifery—and my writing about it—has neither reopened nor foreclosed discussions of the right, best, or most natural way to give birth. Rather, the blog incident speaks to the fundamentally discursive nature of reproductive bodies. In this case, midwifery discourses of nature, tradition, and home inform the identities and practices of midwives and the embodied experiences of women in their care, even as they are persistently shadowed by sometimes hostile, biomedically oriented interlocuters.

If I were to start another study of midwifery today, the issues that would surface most pressingly might be different. Recently announced funding promises from the Ontario provincial government mean that midwifery will grow to account for 20 percent of all births in the province by the year 2020. As midwifery emerges from the margins, other changes are also afoot. A number of long-awaited studies have demonstrated the cost savings of midwifery care compared to physician care. Clinical studies are confirming the safety of planned home births in a system that includes a regulated midwifery profession. Cultural diversity is growing within the professional ranks of midwives and among the clientele. Midwives are facing a new host of professional concerns—legal liability, practice audits, how to assess and incorporate new scientific evidence within one's practice, and how to manage the "caring dilemma" and avoid burnout.

Yet, despite this apparently new terrain, these pressing professional questions are still entangled with the grassroots concerns of midwives to assert the legitimacy of the cultural categories of natural birth, home birth, and women's choice in childbirth. These professional challenges spill over into midwifery knowledge and practice and, in turn, into the spatial and embodied experiences of pregnant and birthing women. But are they contests that unravel the social and political project of midwifery as a radical alternative to "technocratic" birth? Or are they part of its dynamic constitution? Such interpretive and practical debates may be fraught—and they are without a doubt proliferating in some new places, as I discovered—but they are most certainly productive. Midwifery will continue to offer persuasive cultural interventions into nature in the changing context of maternity care in the twenty-first century.

Glossary of Terms and Acronyms

AOM: Association of Ontario Midwives
CHC: community health center
CMM: Committee for More Midwives
CMO: College of Midwives of Ontario
CPSO: College of Physicians and Surgeons of Ontario
HPLR: Health Professions Legislation Review
IMPP: International Midwifery Pre-registration Program
LMCO: Lebel Midwifery Care Organisation
MEP: Midwifery Education Program
MFT-O: Midwifery Task Force of Ontario
MOHLTC: Ministry of Health and Long-Term Care
PLA: Prior Learning Assessment
PLEA: Prior Learning Evaluation and Assessment
OAM: Ontario Association of Midwives
OMCN: Ontario Midwifery Consumers Network
ONMA: Ontario Nurse Midwives' Association
TPA: transfer payment agency
VBAC: vaginal birth after caesarean

Notes

Chapter 1

1. All names of informants have been changed.
2. See Trevathan 1987, 225, for an explanation from the perspective of human evolution for "obligate midwifery."
3. British Columbia and Alberta legalized midwifery in 1998, Manitoba in 2000. Quebec took a slightly different route to professional midwifery, beginning with pilot projects in 1990 which led to midwifery legislation in 1999. Aboriginal midwives have been practicing legally in many places across the country, with notable success in Nunavut and the Northwest Territories for several years. Midwifery legislation is pending in several other provinces.
4. Yanagisako and Delaney (1994) elaborate this idea that social and cultural realities—power differences between men and women, for example, or between groups—are typically given the appearance of being natural and are often underpinned by scientific formulations.
5. Also important in this list is the history of colonial interventions in the name of modernity and civilization, as well as present-day interventions in the name of development.
6. Feminist theory and methods in the social sciences have long been concerned with breaking down the hierarchical relations between the researcher and the researched (Abu-Lughod 1990b; Gluck and Patai 1991; Harding 1987; Stacey 1991; Ong 1995) and with encouraging interested or advocacy positions vis-à-vis the people we study (Stanley and Wise 1990). Indeed, one of the main projects of feminist ethnographers in the

last two decades has been to challenge ethnographic authority based on the premises of objectivity and distance—relations that produce and reproduce a kind of colonial encounter between the ethnographer and his anthropological other/subject (Visweswaran 1994).

7. Though the women in my study shared many visible similarities, they were not an utterly homogeneous group. Their limited diversity was marked by geographic area—some of the concerns of rural women being quite different from those of urban women—as well as age, ethnicity, religion, income, first language. It is also worth noting that in the few years since regulation an increasingly diverse group of women is choosing midwifery.

8. The idea of the midwifery consumer also speaks to the political economy of reproduction in the context of late capitalism and the demographic transition, specifically, the trend toward having fewer children later in life and the trend toward treating pregnancy and childbirth as valuable experiences (Greenhalgh 1995).

9. This effort corresponds to the broader trend in anthropology of acknowledging the collaborative nature of our work and giving voice to the groups and individuals we work with.

10. For example, *Globe and Mail* reporter Alanna Mitchell (1991) called into question the safety of home birth and described it as "anti-woman and anti-child."

11. Goodwin writes in hope that the Atlantic provinces might be spared such "critical error" and recommends that home birth be disallowed. For the ongoing debate about the safety of home birth versus hospital birth in Canada, see Blais 2002, Janssen and Lee 2000, Janssen et al. 2002, Johnson and Davis 2005, and Tyson 1991. For relevant research not limited to Canada, see Anderson and Murphy 1995, Janssen et al. 1994, Olsen and Jewell 2005, and Wiegers et al. 1996. For social science perspectives on the debate, see Bourgeault 1997, Bortin et al. 1994, Campbell and Macfarlane 1994, and Hafner-Eton and Pearce 1994.

12. Meyers-Cieko is the Executive Director of the Seattle Midwifery School. She was speaking about a similar process of exclusion that took place in the political process that led to legal recognition for midwives in the state of Washington.

13. The first midwives in the province were registered through the Michener Institute of Applied Health Sciences in Toronto.

14. *Midwife* became a protected title and practicing midwifery without a license became a criminal offense for the first time.

Chapter 2

1. To a great extent I am focusing my discussion here on historical references regarding Canadian midwifery. For sources on the history of midwifery in the United States specifically, see Donegal 1978, Donnison 1977, Edwards and Waldorf 1984, Ehrenreich and English 1973, Kay 1988, Leavitt 1986, Litoff 1978, Reid 1989, Sullivan and Weitz 1988, Susie 1987, and Wertz and Wertz 1989.

2. The idea of midwifery as a sacred calling may indicate a tendency to exoticize non-Western midwifery while rationalizing European forms.

3. Early obstetricians also redefined the experience of pain along gender and class lines (Sullivan and Weitz 1988, 7). Women were encouraged to think of the pain of childbirth as somehow "uncivilized" and therefore not appropriate for middle and upper class women.

4. In the early part of the twentieth century, the National Council of Women in Canada attempted to set up a program to train and upgrade the skills of experienced neighbor midwives in rural areas. Their efforts were unsuccessful, and nurses were recruited instead to conduct rural deliveries, later becoming the Victorian Order of Nurses. The United Farm Women of Alberta (UFWA) and the United Farm Men of Alberta also lobbied the provincial government during World War I to address the scarcity of physicians and supply midwives to remote areas of the province (Mason 1987). British trained nurse-midwives initially filled such positions but were eventually replaced by local nurses with advanced training in obstetrics.

5. The home birth movement in Canada began on the West Coast (Barrington 1985). For historical and social scientific perspectives on the home birth movement in the United States at this time, see Hosford 1976 and Reid 1989.

6. See, e.g., Odent 1984, Leboyer 1978, Bradley 1974, and Dick-Read 1959.

7. The term *independent* or *lay midwife* is used in the United States to distinguish them from Certified Nurse-Midwives (CNMs) who practice in some states. Lay midwifery is not a term used much in Canada because, as several midwives and commentators have pointed out, the term is inaccurate and often used pejoratively. Midwife and scholar Betty-Ann Daviss notes that midwives in Ontario at this time often referred to themselves as "practicing midwives" to distinguish themselves from nurse-midwives trained in other jurisdictions who were working as obstetric nurses in hospitals (personal communication, 2006). It is also

common now to hear midwives who are not nurses refer to themselves as direct-entry midwives, referring to their educational route to becoming a midwife.

8. The El Paso clinic, *Maternidad de la Luz,* was run by Shari Daniels who, as a speaker during a local home birth conference in the 1980s, issued an open invitation to the Ontario midwifery community to come and train at her clinic, which served a largely migrant Mexican clientele. Sociologist Sheryl Nestel (1996/97, 327) points out the irony in aspiring Ontario midwives traveling across borders to improve their skills on the bodies of "others" and thereby gain their qualifications, while immigrant women of color in Ontario possessing formal qualifications from their countries of origin would not dare to practice outside the law.

9. In 1989, BC midwives Gloria Lemay and Mary Sullivan were convicted of criminal negligence causing death after a home birth where a baby died (Mickelburgh 1990). Their convictions were later overturned. In 1990, after attending a successful home birth, Alberta midwife Noreen Walker was charged with practicing medicine without a license.

10. The ONMA was an interest group because Ontario does not have this professional designation, which is common in many places such as the United Kingdom, the United States, Jamaica, and many African countries. The invitation from the HPLR to midwives seems to acknowledge a number of clear problems with maternity care in the province at that time. Some women were opting out of the system because of the treatment they received in hospitals, and fewer family physicians were doing births because of the disruptions it caused in their family lives and also because of the high cost of malpractice insurance relative to the small number of births they did per year. For a detailed sociological account of the process of midwifery professionalization, see Bourgeault 2006.

11. The first midwifery consumer groups in Canada sprang up in British Columbia in the early 1980s and were the first to propose the idea of securing legislation to regulate midwifery. It was, however, a group of community midwives in Alberta who made the first formal but unsuccessful attempt (Barrington 1985).

12. Vaginal birth after caesarean.

13. See Howarth 1994. Essentially, these experienced, apprentice, or aspiring midwives were given the option of applying to the Midwifery Education program and starting from scratch. Some CMM members did eventually gain their credentials this way, but others did not even gain admission.

14. This definition was jointly developed by the International Confederation

of Midwives and the International Federation of Gynaecology and Obstetrics in the early 1970s. It was later adopted by the World Health Organization. Amended in the early 1990s, it remains the internationally accepted definition.

15. In Alberta, in contrast, midwifery is legal, but clients must pay for it out of pocket as one would for other legitimate but nonlisted medical services such as chiropractic care.

16. Ryerson Polytechnic University, McMaster University, and Laurentian University (which offers the program in French as well as in English).

17. Originally known as the Prior Learning and Assessment (PLA) and later renamed the Prior Learning and Experience Assessment (PLEA), this program was instituted only after a period of lobbying by the CMM. The first group graduated through the PLA in the fall of 1996 and became Registered Midwives.

18. See Couchie and Nabigon 1998 and Carroll and Benoit 2004 for descriptions of Aboriginal midwifery across Canada.

19. See Nestel 2004 on foreign-trained and immigrant women of color "excluded" by midwifery professionalization.

20. Media coverage of an inquest into a neonatal death in Guelph, Ontario, in 2001 noted that the relationships between midwives and OBs, pediatricians, and nurses at the Guelph General Hospital were *"terrible"*— not simply a case of growing pains. The dysfunctional institutional culture of the hospital was seen to be the root of the problem. It was further noted that this situation was not isolated to Guelph. The jury went so far as to recommend that action be taken by Guelph General Hospital to improve communication between doctors, nurses, and midwives. See Bruce 2001 and also Shuttleworth 2002.

21. The Ontario Ministry of Health and Long Term Care (MOHLTC) undertook a review in 2003 which found that midwifery was not only cost effective but was cost saving for the provincial health care system (AOM 2007a). The savings derive from a number of factors. First, normal births are not handled by specialists whose services cost more. Second, home births do not require the use of hospital beds and services such as meals and housekeeping. Third, planned hospital birth clients usually leave the hospital sooner because midwives provide follow-up postpartum care at home—a feature of midwifery which also translates into lower hospital and emergency room readmission rates. Fourth, midwifery is associated with less technology and medication during labor as well as lower rates of interventions generally (Johnson and Daviss 2005). For example, when

compared to family physicians with a comparable group of low risk cases, midwives have lower rates of episiotomy (7.2 vs. 16.6%), forceps/ vacuum deliveries (5.4 vs. 14.4%), and referrals to caesarean section (12.7 vs. 20.6%). The Ministry report also found that midwifery had very high client satisfaction rates (98.7%) and good clinical outcomes with maternal and infant mortality and morbidity rates being comparable to national rates of all births and rates of family physicians following a comparable cohort of low risk cases (AOM 2007b); Kaufman et al. 2001a; Kaufman et al. 2001b). It is also worth noting that midwifery clients had higher rates of breastfeeding uptake and continuation at six weeks postpartum (90.7%) compared to those in physician care (71.5%) (AOM 2007b).

22. Very rarely will a client request care outside midwifery standards of practice. For example, a woman may refuse an intervention or refuse to give birth in a hospital even though she has a condition that is contraindicated for home birth or midwifery care. If this occurs in advance of the onset of labor, the CMO directs midwives to advise the woman of the risks, take steps to transfer the care, and protect themselves legally (by sending a registered letter to the woman's home outlining what has been communicated in clinic). In the event that a woman still does not accept a transfer of care, especially if this happens while labor is underway, the midwife should provide care while continuing to advise her of the risks.

Chapter 3

1. Several other works addressing specific topics fill out this list, including Nancy Wainer Cohen's *The Silent Knife* (1982) on C-sections, and *Open Season* on vaginal birth after caesarean (1991). Aspiring midwives also studied clinical manuals and textbooks.

2. The political rhetoric of the popular and scholarly alternative childbirth literature was highly oppositional during this time. See Barrington 1985; Kitzinger 1988; Rothman 1982.

3. See also Kitzinger's other works: *The Place of Birth* (with John Davis, 1978), *Birth at Home* (1980), and *Home Birth: The Essential Guide to Giving Birth outside the Hospital* (1982).

4. Certainly, things have improved since the 1980s when this study was carried out. Pubic-area shaving and enemas are no longer routine everywhere; many hospitals now have labor, delivery, and recovery rooms

(LDRs); some hospitals have birthing suites with baths and instruments tucked out of sight behind curtains and cupboards. Several scientific studies have demonstrated the detrimental overuse of episiotomies and C-sections, and some physicians and hospital have listened. Some feminist critics and activists, however, describe such changes as little more than cosmetic, the belated co-optation of the natural birth movement. Meanwhile, pharmaceutical interventions continue routinely, and C-section rates remain high.

5. Birthing chairs and ropes, for example, are now part of alternative birthing technology in midwifery in places like Ontario.

6. See also Bradley 1974 and Leboyer 1978.

7. See, e.g., Griffin 1978; Merchant 1983; and Shiva 1988. Critiques of this perspective characterize it as an appropriation that serves Western projects through the erasure of difference between Western and non-Western people and a false objectification of indigenous identity as statically premodern. Geographer Jane Jacobs, however, argues that sometimes such "imaginative projections" about people in other times and places can become powerful political rallying points around which both Western and non-Western goals may be achieved (1994, 190). A handful of midwives registered in Ontario and Quebec, for example, are deeply involved with training programs for Inuit midwives in the far North of Canada, in the territory of Nunavut.

8. Chapters in this edited volume explicitly link midwifery with the everyday knowledge of women as mothers. William Wedenoja, for example, in his essay on healing in Jamaica, suggests that nurturance—"the mothering element of healing"—is a cultural universal (1989, 76–77).

9. While Catherine Reissman (1983), for example, has described how middle- and upper-class women colluded with physicians in the goal of pain-free childbirth or "twilight sleep," the medicalization of pregnancy and childbirth has become so thorough and routinized as to make this statement generally indisputable.

10. See also Kay et al. 1988 and Sullivan and Weitz 1988, who address internal divisions within midwifery from the perspective of midwives as workers, showing their concerns as sometimes incompatible with the model of midwifery care.

11. According to the *Chamber's Dictionary, empower* means "to authorize" and *empowerment* means "the giving to individuals of the power to

take decisions in matters relating to themselves" (1993, 550). The term *empowerment* as it is used in midwifery discourse also conveys the sense of feeling powerful, strong, and capable.

12. The political divide between midwives who identify themselves as pro-choice or pro-life is more pronounced in the United States than in Canada.

13. The importance of midwifery being about reproductive choices for women was made clear again quite recently in Toronto. Due to massive hospital restructuring in the city, some midwives were forced to move their privileges to a Catholic hospital, which had so far been without midwives. While their reluctance to practice in the Catholic hospital is, in part, a workplace issue for midwives who will have to reestablish themselves in a new environment, some are also concerned that they will not be able to offer women real reproductive choices in such an environment.

14. See, e.g., Barrington 1985; James-Chetalet 1989; Mason 1987; and Shroff 1997.

15. "Midwife: A Heritage Minute" is one of several dozen vignettes produced by Heritage Canada that depict important events and characters in Canadian society and history. For a longer description and analysis of the vignette, see MacDonald 2004.

16. That the practice of women helping women in childbirth is ancient and near universal is an assertion about which there can be little debate. See Wenda Trevathan for an explanation of "obligate midwifery" from the perspective biological anthropology (1987).

17. *Doula* is the name given to the person who cares for the new mother after childbirth and who may also assist at the birth. It is an informal but important role, usually taken on by close female relatives, neighbors, and friends who provide support for successful early mothering, especially breastfeeding (Raphael 1966). Since the 1980s some women have offered doula services for a fee or barter, and doula training programs and professional associations now exist in Canada and the United States.

18. See Marchand and Parpart (1995) and Pigg (1997) for critical discussions of this tendency.

19. *Midwifery birth culture* and *alternative birth culture* are terms I heard often over the course of this study. They refer to an array of knowledge and practices that extend beyond pregnancy and birth to include nutrition, health, spirituality, and environmentalism, as well as social and relational values. Midwifery birth culture is a powerful legitimizing notion

that highlights the will of its members to promote and protect it, and also reflects the increasing imperative for midwives to engage in self-representation.

20. For example, the granny midwives in her study address postpartum hemorrhage by raising the foot of the bed while chanting and praying (1978, 163).

21. This is not to say that midwives resist change of all kinds. Indeed, traditional midwives welcome many changes. Brigitte Jordan (1993), for example, tells the story of how several Mexican *parteras* with whom she worked stopped telling women to push "too soon" after her suggestion that women could be allowed to wait for a time between the second and third stages of labor without harming mother or infant.

22. See Klassen 2001 for a discussion of the relationship between religion and home birth.

23. Petra is referring to one of several incidents that took place the 1980s in which women gathered on the steps of the Manulife Centre in a posh shopping and banking district of Toronto after a woman was asked to leave for breastfeeding her infant in public. They breastfed their infants to make the point that breastfeeding in public should be accepted.

24. Several midwives and women I spoke to indicated to me that there may be home births happening outside the system.

Chapter 4

1. Throughout this chapter and elsewhere in the book, I do not use quotes around the word natural (for the sake of elegance), but it should be clear to the reader that I am critically deconstructing the term as it is used in contemporary midwifery.

2. Midwives argue that natural birth is empowering for families, too, in various ways, for example, allowing fathers, other children, and even grandparents a greater role in the process.

3. A condition that occurs during pregnancy or during labor in which the placenta pulls away from the uterus, causing bleeding and an emergency situation.

4. Heather Paxson's article "Rationalising Risk."

5. Low hemoglobin levels may lead to anemia, which, if severe, can cause complications during pregnancy and delivery.

6. Gestational age upon which the due date is calculated may be "confirmed" several times during pregnancy with different results each

time. It is not uncommon for women to have their dates moved back and forth two or three times during pregnancy.

7. Some scholars further posit that it is men's profound alienation from reproduction which underscores their desire to master and control it through the mastery and control of women (O'Brien 1981). They argue that the example of new reproductive and genetic technologies are the most recent manifestation of this tendency (Corea 1985; Overall 1987).

8. Maternal serum is a screening test performed at fifteen to eighteen weeks of pregnancy and is used to signal maternal risk for several fetal disabilities including neural tube disorders and Down Syndrome. It is not a diagnostic test, and thus critics suggest that it creates anxiety and leads to increased use of other technologies (Blatt 1993, 237).

9. At the time I conducted the research for this book in the late 1990s, midwives attended approximately 6 percent of all births in the province; that figure had risen to 8 percent by 2007.

10. Meconium is the first stool excreted by the infant. Interuterine excretion (which can only be detected after the amniotic waters have broken) is associated with fetal distress. Meconium aspiration is a potentially dangerous situation for the baby and requires hospital-based intervention (Raines 1993, 244).

11. Back labor, said to cause the worst kind of labor pain, is so called because it describes the position of the baby pressing on a woman's spine during labor.

12. How midwifery and home birth affect the partners of birthing women is an important and interesting topic, but I do not elaborate on it here.

Chapter 5

1. The percentage of home births in Ontario has declined slowly since legalization from approximately 50 percent of all midwifery clients in 1993 (Van Wagner 2005) to between 20 and 25 percent in 2006 (Knox and Katherine 2007).

2. For a detailed account and legal analysis of the creation and demise of the Toronto Birth Centre, see Sutton 1996.

3. Sociologist Daniel Miller's work on how the use of objects in the home become part of personal and collective identity building is an important exception to this infatuation with large-scale and public phenomena. Anthropologists Janelle Taylor, Lynda Layne, and Danielle Wosniak have also edited a volume of papers on the relationships between domestic

scale consumption and the display of everyday objects in homes and
workplaces in the construction of mothers and fetuses as particular kinds
of persons in the age of late capitalism (2004).

4. See Chapter 1, note 11 for the ongoing debate about the safety of home
   birth versus hospital birth in Canada and elsewhere.

5. This is not always the case. Some women labor well whether other
   people are there or not. The difference, according to midwives, can be a
   woman's level of confidence and self-assuredness. I have attended several
   births involving a small group of friends and heard stories of others
   involving a near crowd of friends and relatives. In one particularly unique
   case a woman labored and gave birth downstairs with a video camera on,
   projecting the image to a TV upstairs where more than a dozen of her
   family and friends watched and waited.

6. See note 1.

7. This process of rethinking the body starts well before labor. Like most
   midwives, Jackie took every opportunity to convey to her clients her
   view of women's bodies as perfectly suited to carry pregnancies and give
   birth. At prenatal visits she reminded women that they had "lots of room
   down there!"

References Cited

Abu-Lughod, Lila. 1990a. "The Romance of Resistance: Tracing Transformations of Power through Bedouin Women." *American Ethnologist* 17 (1): 44–55.

——— 1990b. "Can There Be A Feminist Ethnography?" *Women and Performance* 5 (1): 1–27.

Adelson, Naomi. 2000. *Being Alive Well: Health and the Politics of Cree Well-Being.* Toronto: University of Toronto Press.

Allen, Denise Roth. 2003. *Managing Motherhood, Managing Risk.* Ann Arbor: University of Michigan Press.

Anderson, R., and P. Murphy. 1995. "Outcomes of 11,788 Planned Home Births Attended by Certified Nurse-Midwives." *Journal of Nurse Midwifery* 6:483–92.

Arms, Suzanne. 1975. *Immaculate Deception.* New York: Bantam.

Association of Ontario Midwives. 2007a. "Benefits of Midwifery to the Health Care System." Available at www.aom.on.ca (accessed April 15, 2007).

———. 2007b. "Benefits to Women Needing Obstetrical Care: A Case for Sustaining Midwifery." Available at www.aom.on.ca (accessed April 15, 2007).

Bachelard, Gaston. 1958. *The Poetics of Space.* Boston: Beacon.

Barrington, Elizabeth. 1985. *Midwifery is Catching.* Toronto: New Canada Publishers.

Benoit, Cecilia. 1987. "Uneasy Partners: Midwives and Their Clients." *Canadian Journal of Sociology* 12:275–84.

———. 1991. *Midwives in Passage.* St. John's, Newfoundland: Institute of Social and Economic Research.

Berdoulay, Vincent. 1986. "Place, Meaning, and Discourse in French Language Geography." In *The Power of Place*, ed. J. Agnew and J. Duncan, 124–39. London: Unwin Hyman.

Berthelot, J. M. 1984. "Sociological Discourse and the Body." *Theory, Culture, and Society* 3 (3): 155–64.

Biggs, Leslie. 1983. "The Case of the Missing Midwives: A History of Midwifery in Ontario from 1795-1900." *Ontario History* 75:21–35.

———. 2004. "Rethinking the History of Midwifery in Canada." In *Reconceiving Midwifery*, ed. Bourgeault, Benoit, and Davis-Floyd, 17–45.

Blais, Régis. 2002. "Are Home Births Safe?" *Canadian Medical Association Journal* 166 (3): 335–36.

Blatt, R. J. 1993. "Maternal Serum Screening." In *The Encyclopedia of Childbearing*, ed. Rothman, 236–37.

Blunt, Alison, and Gillian Rose, eds. 1994. *Writing Women and Space*. New York: Guilford.

Boddy, Janice. 1995. "Managing Tradition: 'Superstition' and the Making of National Identity among Sudanese Women Refugees." In *The Pursuit of Certainty: Religious and Cultural Formations*, ed. W. James, 17–44. London: Routledge.

Bortin, S., et al. 1994. "A Feminist Perspective on the Study of Home Birth." *Journal of Nurse Midwifery* 39 (3): 142–49.

Bourdieu, Pierre. 1977. *Outline of a Theory of Practice*. Cambridge: Cambridge University Press.

Bourgeault, Ivy Lynn. 1996. "Delivering Midwifery: An Examination of the Process and Outcome of Regulating Midwifery in Ontario." Ph.D. thesis, University of Toronto.

———. 1997. "The Safety of Home Birth: A Review of the Literature." Unpublished report prepared for York University Centre for Health Studies.

———. 2006. *Push!* Toronto: McGill-Queen's University Press.

Bourgeault, Ivy Lynn, Cecilia Benoit, and Robbie Davis-Floyd, eds. 2004. *Reconceiving Midwifery*. Montreal: McGill-Queens University Press.

Bradley, Robert. 1974. *Husband-Coached Childbirth*. New York: Harper and Row.

Bruce, Andrew. 2001. "Midwives, MDs Urged to Cooperate; Baby Death Inquest Calls for Change." *Toronto Star*. December 6.

Burtch, Brian. 1988. "Midwifery and the State: The New Midwifery in Canada." In *Gender and Society: Creating a Canadian Women's Sociology*, ed. A. Mclaren, 349–77. Toronto: Pitman.

———— 1994. *The Trials of Labour.* Montreal: McGill-Queens University Press.

Butler, Judith. 1990. *Gender Trouble.* New York: Routledge.

———— 1993. *Bodies That Matter.* New York: Routledge.

Campanella, Karla, Jill Korbin, and Louise Acheson. 1993. "Pregnancy and Childbirth among the Amish." *Social Science and Medicine* 36 (3): 333–42.

Campbell, R., and A. Macfarlane. 1994. *Where to be Born?: The Debate and the Evidence.* Oxford: National Perinatal Epidemiology Unit.

Carroll, Dena, and Cecilia Benoit. 2004. "Aboriginal Midwifery in Canada." In *Reconceiving Midwifery,* ed. Bourgeault, Benoit, and Davis-Floyd, 263–86.

Cohen, Nancy Wainer. 1991. *Open Season: A Survival Guide for Natural Childbirth and VBAC in the 1990s.* New York: Bergin and Garvey.

Cohen, Nancy Wainer, and Lois Estner. 1982. *Silent Knife: Cesarean Prevention and Vaginal Birth after Cesarean.* New York: Bergin and Garvey.

College of Physicians and Surgeons of Ontario. 1982. *Statement on Home Birth.*

Comaroff, Jean. 1995. *Body of Power, Spirit of Resistance.* Chicago: University of Chicago Press.

Corea, Gena. 1985. *The Mother Machine.* New York: Harper and Row.

Cosminsky, Sheila. 1976. "Cross-Cultural Perspectives on Midwifery." In *Medical Anthropology,* ed. X. Francis, S. Grollig, and H. Hatley, 229–48. The Hague: Mouton.

———— 1977. "Childbirth and Midwifery on a Guatemalan Finca." *Medical Anthropology* 6 (3): 69–104.

Couchie, Carol, and Herbert Nabigon. 1998. "A Path Towards Reclaiming Nishnawbe Birth Culture: Can the Midwifery Exemption Clause make a Difference?" In *The New Midwifery,* ed. Shroff, 41–50.

Davis-Floyd, Robbie. 1992. *Birth As an American Rite of Passage.* Berkeley: University of California Press.

————. 1994. "The Technocratic Body: American Childbirth as Cultural Expression." *Social Science and Medicine* 38 (8): 1125–40.

Davis-Floyd, Robbie, and Carolyn Sargent, eds. 1997. *Childbirth and Authoritative Knowledge.* Berkeley: University of California Press.

Davis-Floyd, Robbie, and Elizabeth Davis. 1997. "Intuition as Authoritative Knowledge in Midwifery and Homebirth." In *Childbirth and Authoritative Knowledge,* ed. Davis-Floyd and Sargent, 315–49.

Daviss, Betty Anne. 2001. "Reforming Birth and Remaking Midwifery in North America." In *Birth by Design,* ed. DeVries, Benoit, Van Teijlingen, and Wrede, 70–86.

DeVries, Ray, Cecilia Benoit, Edwin Van Teijlingen, and Sirpa Wrede. 2001.

Birth by Design: Pregnancy, Maternity Care and Midwifery in North America and Europe. London: Routledge.

DeVries, Raymond, and Rebecca Barosso. 1997. "Midwives among the machines." In *Midwives, Society and Childbirth: Debates and Controversies in the Modern Period*, ed. Hilary Marland. London: Routledge.

Dick-Read, Grantley. 1959. *Childbirth Without Fear.* New York: Harper and Row.

Di Giacomo, Susan. 1987. "Biomedicine as a Cultural System: An Anthropologist in the Kingdom of the Sick." In *Encounters with Biomedicine*, ed. H. Baer, 315–46. Montreux: Gordon and Breach Science Publishers.

Donegal, Jean. 1978. *Women and Men Midwives: Medicine, Morality, and Misogyny in Early America.* Westport, CT: Greenwood Press.

Donnison, Jean. 1977. *Midwives and Medical Men: A History of Intra-Professional Rivalries and Women's Rights.* New York: Schocken.

Dougherty, Molly. 1978. "Southern Lay Midwives as Ritual Specialists." In *Women in Ritual and Symbolic Roles,* ed. J. Hoch-Smith and A. Spring, 151–64. New York: Plenum.

Duden, Barbara. 1991. *The Woman Beneath the Skin.* Trans. Thomas Dunlop. Cambridge: Harvard University Press.

Duncan, Nancy, ed. 1996. *BodySpace.* London: Routledge.

Edwards, Margot, and Mary Waldorf. 1984. *Reclaiming Birth: History and Heroines of American Childbirth Reform.* New York: Crossing Press.

Ehrenreich, Barbara, and Deirdre English. 1973. *Witches, Midwives, and Nurses: A History of Women Healers.* Old Westbury, NY: Feminist Press.

——— 1978. *For Her Own Good.* New York: Doubleday.

Emad, Mitra. 1996. "Twirling the Needle: Pinning Down Anthropologists' Emergent Bodies in the Disclosive Field of American Acupuncture." Paper presented at the American Anthropological Association Annual Meeting, Washington, DC.

Firestone, Shulamith. 1972. *The Dialectic of Sex.* London: Paladin.

Foucault, Michel. 1975. *The Birth of the Clinic.* New York: Vintage.

——— 1977. *Discipline and Punish.* New York: Vintage.

——— 1980a. *The History of Sexuality.* New York: Vintage.

——— 1980b. "The Eye of Power." In *Power/Knowledge,* 146–49. New York: Pantheon.

Fraser, Gertrude. 1995. "Modern Bodies, Modern Minds: Midwifery and Reproductive Change in an African American Community." In *Conceiving the New World Order,* ed. Ginsburg and Rapp, 42–58.

Gallagher, Catherine, and Thomas Laqueur, eds. 1987. *The Making of the Modern Body.* Berkeley: University of California Press.

Gaskin, Ina May. 1989. *Spiritual Midwifery.* Summertown, PA: Book Publishing Company.

Ginsburg, F., and A. Lowenhaupt-Tsing, eds. 1990. *Uncertain Terms: Negotiating Gender in American Culture.* Boston: Beacon.

Ginsburg, Faye, and Rayna Rapp, eds. 1995. *Conceiving the New World Order.* Berkeley: University of California Press.

Gluck, Sherna Berger, and Daphne Patai. 1991. *Women's Words.* New York: Routledge.

Goodwin, James. 1997. "Where to Be Born Safely: Professional Midwifery and the Case Against Home Birth." *Journal of the Society of Obstetricians and Gynaecologists of Canada* 19 (11): 1179–88.

Greenhalgh, Susan, ed. 1995. *Situating Fertility.* London: Cambridge University Press.

Griffin, Susan. 1978. *Woman and Nature: The Roaring Within Her.* New York: Perennial.

Gupta, Akhil, and James Ferguson. 1992. "Beyond 'Culture': Space, Identity, and the Politics of Difference." *Cultural Anthropology* 7 (1): 6–23.

Hafner-Eaton, C., and L. K. Pearce. 1994. "Birth Choices, the Law, and Medicine: Balancing Individual Freedoms and the Protection of the Public's Health." *Journal of Health Politics, Policy and Law* 19 (4): 813–35.

Handler, Richard, and Jocelyn Linnekin. 1984. "Tradition, Genuine and Spurious." *Journal of American Folklore* 97:273–90.

Hanson, Allan. 1989. "The Making of the Maori: Cultural Invention and Its Logic." *American Anthropologist* 91 (4): 890–902.

Haraway, Donna. 1991. *Simians, Cyborgs, and Women.* New York: Routledge.

Harding, Sandra. 1987. *Feminism and Methodology.* Bloomington: Indiana University Press.

Hartmann, K., and M. Viswanathan, R. Palmieri, G. Gartlehner, J. Thorp Jr., and K. L. Lohr. 2005. "Outcomes of Routine Episiotomy: A Systematic Review." *JAMA* 293:2141–48.

Hoch-Smith, Judith, and Anita Spring, eds. 1978. *Women in Ritual and Symbolic Roles.* New York: Plenum.

hooks, bell. 1990. *Yearning: Race, Gender, and Cultural Politics.* Boston: South End.

Hosford, Elisabeth. 1976. "The Home Birth Movement." *Journal of Nurse-Midwifery* 21 (3): 27–30.

Howarth, Leslie. 1994. "Another Side to Midwifery Legislation in Ontario." *Aspiring Midwife* 5:21–23.

Jacobs, Jane. 1994. "Earth Honoring: Western Desires and Indigenous Knowledges." In *Writing Women and Space,* ed. Blunt and Rose, 169–96.

James-Chetalet, Lois. 1989. "Reclaiming the Birth Experience: An Analysis of Midwifery in Canada from 1788 to 1987." Ph.D. diss., Carleton University.

Janssen, P. A., V. L. Hold, and S. J. Meyers. 1994. "Licensed Midwife-Attended Out-of-Hospital Births in Washington State: Are They Safe?" *Birth* 21(3): 141–48.

Janssen, P., and S. Lee. 2000. "Home Birth Demonstration Project. Final Report to the Health Transition Fund." Project no BC404. Victoria: British Columbia Ministry of Health and Ministry Responsible for Seniors.

Janssen, Patricia A., Shoo K. Lee, Elizabeth M. Ryan, Duncan J. Etches, Duncan F. Farquharson, Donlim Peacock, and Michael C. Klein. 2002. "Outcomes of Planned Home Births Versus Planned Hospital Births After Regulation of Midwifery in British Columbia." *CMAJ* 166 (3): 315–23.

Jeffery, Patricia, Roger Jeffery, and Andrew Lyon. 1989. *Labour Pains and Labour Power: Women and Childbearing in India.* London: Zed.

Jezioranski, Lisa. 1987. "Towards a New Status for the Midwifery Profession in Ontario." *McGill Law Journal* 33:90–136.

Johnson, K., and B. A. Daviss. 2005. "Outcomes of Planned Home Births with Certified Professional Midwives: Large Prospective Study in North America." *BMJ* 330: 1416–21.

Jordan, Brigitte. 1987. "The Hut and the Hospital: Information, Power, and Symbolism in the Artifacts of Birth." *Birth* 14 (1): 36–40.

———. 1993 [1978]. *Birth in Four Cultures.* Prospect Heights, IL: Waveland.

Kahn, Susan Martha. 2000. *Reproducing Jews.* Durham: Duke University Press.

Kanaaneh, Rhoda Ann. 2002. *Birthing the Nation. Strategies of Palestinian Women in Israel.* Berkeley: University of California Press.

Kaufert, Patricia, and John O'Neill. 1993. "Analysis of a Dialogue on Risk in Childbirth: Clinicians, Epidemiologists, and Inuit Women." In *Knowledge, Power, and Practice: The Anthropology of Medicine and Everyday Life,* ed. S. Lindenbaum and M. Lock, 32–54. Berkeley: University of California Press.

Kaufman, K., J. Honigbirk, R. Pong, and L. Martin. 2001a. "Midwifery Care in Ontario: Client Outcomes for 1998, Part 1: Maternal Outcomes." *Ontario Midwives Journal* 7 (2): 56–64.

————. 2001b. "Midwifery Care in Ontario: Client Outcomes for 1998, Part 2: Fetal and Newborn Outcomes." *AOM Journal* 7 (4): 147–53.

Kaufman, Karen, and Bobbi Soderstrom. 2004. "Midwifery Education in Ontario." In *Reconceiving Midwifery,* ed. Bourgeault, Benoit, and Davis-Floyd, 187–203.

Kay, Bonnie, et al. 1988. "Women's Health and Social Change: The Case of Lay Midwives." *International Journal of Health Services* 18 (2): 223–35.

Kay, Margarita. 1982. *Anthropology of Human Birth.* Philadelphia: F. A. Davis.

Keesing, Roger. 1982. "Kastom and Anticolonialism on Malaita: 'Culture' as Political Symbol." *Mankind* 13 (4): 357–73.

Kitzinger, Sheila. 1980. *Birth at Home.* New York: Viking Penguin.

————. 1982. *Home Birth: The Essential Guide to Giving Birth Outside the Hospital.* New York: Dorling Kindersley.

————, ed. 1988. *The Midwife Challenge.* London: Pandora.

Kitzinger, Sheila, and John Davis, eds. 1978. *The Place of Birth.* London: Oxford University Press.

Klassen, Pamela. 2001. *Blessed Events.* Princeton: Princeton University Press.

Klaus, Marshall, et al. 1986. "Effects of Social Support During Parturition on Maternal and Infant Morbidity." *British Medical Journal* 293:585–87.

Kleinman, Arthur. 1988. *The Illness Narratives.* New York: Basic Books.

Knox, S., and W. Katherine. 2006. Ontario Midwifery Clinical Data Base. Available at www.apheo.ca/events/06/conf06/W_Catherine_S_Knox_ MidwiferyDatabase.pdf (accessed April 15, 2007).

Kornelsen, Jude, and Elaine Carty. 2004. "Challenges to Midwifery Integration: Interprofessional Relationships in British Columbia." In *Reconceiving Midwifery,* ed. Bourgeault, Benoit, and Davis-Floyd, 111–30.

Laderman, Carol. 1983. *Wives and Midwives.* Berkeley: University of California Press.

Laforce, Helene. 1990. "The Different Stages of the Elimination of Midwives in Quebec." *Delivering Motherhood: Maternal Ideologies and Practices in the 19th and 20th Centuries,* ed. K. Arnup, A. Levesque, and R. Pierson, 36–50. London: Routledge.

Lang, Raven. 1972. *Birth Book.* Ben Lomond, CA: Genesis.

Leavitt, Judith. 1986. *Brought to Bed: Childbearing in America, 1750–1950.* New York: Oxford University Press.

Leboyer, Frederick. 1978. *Birth Without Violence.* New York: Alfred Knopf.

Litoff, Judy Barret. 1978. *American Midwives: 1860 to the Present.* Westport, CT: Greenwood Press.

Livingstone, Martha. 1993. "Read Method: Natural Childbirth." In *The Encyclopedia of Childbearing,* ed. Rothman, 347–48.

Lock, Margaret. 1993. "Cultivating the Body: Anthropology and Epistemologies of Bodily Practice and Knowledge." *Annual Review of Anthropology* 22:133–55.

Lock, Margaret, and Nancy Scheper-Hughes. 1990. "A Critical Interpretive Approach in Medical Anthropology: Rituals and Routines of Discipline and Dissent." In *Medical Anthropology: Contemporary Theory and Method,* ed. T. Johnson and C. Sargent, 47–72. New York: Greenwood.

Lock, Margaret, and Patricia Kaufert, eds. 1998. *Pragmatic Women and Body Politics.* Cambridge: Cambridge University Press.

MacCormack, Carol, ed. 1982. *Ethnography of Fertility and Birth.* New York: Academic Press.

MacDonald, Margaret. 1994. "Reading Disorder: An Illness Narrative in Anthropology." *Sante/Culture/Health* 10 (1–2): 61–81.

——— 2004. "Tradition as a Political Symbol in the New Midwifery in Canada." In *Reconceiving Midwifery,* ed. Bourgeault, Benoit, and Davis-Floyd, 46–66. Montreal and Kingston: McGill-Queens University Press.

MacDonald, Margaret, and Ivy Lynn Bourgeault. 2000. "The Politics of Representation: Doing and Writing Interested Research on Midwifery." *Resources for Feminist Research* 28 (1–2): 151–68.

Marchand, Marianne, and Jane Parpart, eds. *Feminism/Postmodernism/Development.* London: Routledge.

Martin, Biddy, and Chandra Talpade Mohanty. 1986. "Feminist Politics: What's Home Got to Do with it?" In *Feminist Studies/Critical Studies*, ed. T. de Lauretis, 191–212. Bloomington: University of Indiana Press.

Martin, Emily. 1987. *The Woman in the Body.* Boston: Beacon Press.

———. 1991. "The Egg and the Sperm: How Science Has Created a Romance Based on Stereotypical Male-Female Roles." *Signs* 16 (3): 485–501.

———. 1992. "The End of the Body?" *American Ethnologist* 19 (1): 120–38.

Mason, Jutta. 1987. "The History of Midwifery in Canada." In *Report of the Task Force on the Implementation of Midwifery in Ontario,* ed. M. Eberts, A. Schwartz, R. Edney, and K. Kaufman. Toronto: Queen's Park.

———. 1990. *The Trouble with Licensing Midwives.* Ottawa: CRIAW/ICREF.

McClain, Carol. 1975. "Ethno-Obstetrics in Ajijic." *Anthropological Quarterly* 48 (1): 38–56.

———. 1981. "Traditional Midwives and Family Planning." *Medical Anthropology* 5:107–36.

————. 1982. "Towards a Comparative Framework for the Study of Childbirth." In *Anthropology of Human Birth,* ed. M. Kay, 25–59. Philadelphia: F. A. Davis.

————, ed. 1989. *Women as Healers.* New Brunswick: Rutgers University Press.

Mead, Margaret. 1972. *Blackberry Winter: My Early Years.* New York: William Morrow.

Merchant, Carolyn. 1983. *The Death of Nature.* New York: Harper Collins.

Michaelson, Karen, ed. 1988. *Childbirth in America: Anthropological Perspectives.* New York: Bergin and Garvey.

Michie, Helene, and Naomi Cahn. 2000. "Unnatural Births: Cesarean Sections in the Discourse of the 'Natural Childbirth Movement.'" In *Gender and Health,* ed. Carolyn Sargent and Caroline Brettell, 44–56. Upper Saddle River, NJ: Prentice Hall.

Mickleburgh, Rod. 1988. "Case Renews Long-Standing Debate." *Toronto Globe and Mail,* November 13.

Miller, Daniel. 1997. "How Infants Grow Mothers in North London." *Theory, Culture and Society* 14 (4): 76–88.

Mitchell, Alanna. 1991. "Never Mind the Lovely Experience." *Toronto Globe and Mail,* May 3.

Mitchell, Lisa. 1994. "The Routinization of the Other: Ultrasound, Women, and the Fetus." In *Misconceptions,* vol. 2, ed. G. Basen, M. Eichler, and A. Lipman, 146–60. Hull: Voyageuer.

Mitchenson, Wendy. 1991. *The Nature of Their Bodies: Women and Their Doctors in Victorian Canada.* Toronto: University of Toronto Press.

————. 2002. *Giving Birth in Canada, 1900–1950.* Toronto: University of Toronto Press.

Moore, Henrietta. 1986. *Space, Text, and Gender.* Cambridge: Cambridge University Press.

Narayan, Kirin. 1997. "How Native is a Native Anthropologist?" In *Situated Lives: Gender and Culture in Everyday Life,* ed. L. Lamphere, H. Ragone, and P. Zavella. New York: Routledge.

Nestel, Sheryl. 1996–97. "A New Profession to the White Population in Canada: Ontario Midwifery and the Politics of Race." *Health and Canadian Society* 4 (1): 315–41.

————. 1995. "Other Mothers: Race and Representation in Natural Childbirth Discourse." *Resources for Feminist Research* 23 (4): 5–19.

————. 2006. *Obstructed Labour: Race and Gender in the Re-Emergence of Midwifery.* Vancouver: University of British Columbia Press.

Oakley, Anne. 1984. *The Captured Womb: A History of the Medical Care of Pregnant Women.* Oxford: Basil Blackwell.

O'Brien, Mary. 1981. *The Politics of Reproduction.* London: Routledge and Kegan Paul.

Odent, Michel. *Birth Reborn.* New York: Pantheon.

Olsen. O., and M. D. Jewell. 2005. "Home Versus Hospital Births." *Cochrane Database of Systematic Review.* 4.

O'Neill, John, and Patricia Kaufert. 1990. "The Politics of Obstetric Care: The Inuit Experience." In *Births and Social Change,* ed. P. Handwerker, 53–68. Boulder: Westview.

Ong, Aihwa. 1995. "Women out of China: Traveling Tales and Traveling Theories in Postcolonial Feminism." In *Women Writing Culture*, ed. R. Behar and D. Gordon. Berkeley: University of California Press, 350–72.

Oudshoorn, Nelly. 1994. *Beyond the Natural Body.* London: Routledge.

Overall, Christine. 1987. *Ethics and Human Reproduction.* Winchester, MA: Allen and Unwin.

Pasveer, Bernike, and Madeleine Akrich. 2001. "Obstetrical Trajectories: On Training Women's Bodies for (Home)Birth." In *Birth by Design,* ed. DeVries, Benoit, Van Teijlingen, and Wrede, 229–42.

Paxson, Heather. 2002. "Rationalising Sex: Family Planning and the Making of Modern Lovers in Urban Greece." *American Ethnologist* 29 (2): 307–34.

Peterson, Karen. 1992. "Technology as a Last Resort in Homebirth: The Work of Lay Midwives." *Social Problems* 30 (3): 272–83.

Pigg, Stacey Leigh. 1997. "Authority in Translation: Finding, Knowing, Naming 'Traditional Birth Attendants' in Nepal." In *Childbirth and Authoritative Knowledge,* ed. Davis-Floyd and Sargent, 233–62.

Plummer, Kate. 2000. "From Nursing Outpost to Contemporary Midwifery in Canada." *Journal of Midwifery and Women's Health* 45 (2): 169–75.

Rabinow, Paul, ed. 1984. *The Foucault Reader.* New York: Pantheon.

Raines, Deborah. 1993. "Meconium." In *The Encyclopedia of Childbearing,* ed. Rothman, 243–44.

Ram, Kalpana, and Margaret Jolly, eds. 1998. *Maternities and Modernities.* London: Cambridge University Press.

Raphael, Dana. 1993. "Doula." In *The Encyclopedia of Childbearing,* ed. Rothman, 113–15.

Rapp, Rayna. 1990. "Constructing Amniocentesis: Maternal and Medical Discourses." In *Uncertain Terms,* ed. Ginsburg and Lowenhaupt-Tsing, 28–42.

———. 1991. "Moral Pioneers: Men, Women, and Fetuses on a Frontier of

Reproductive Technology." In *Gender at the Crossroads of Knowledge,* ed.
  M. di Leonardo, 383–96. Berkeley: University of California Press.
Reid, Margaret. 1989. "Sisterhood and Professionalization: A Case Study of the
  American Lay Midwife." In *Women as Healers,* ed. C. McClain, 219–38.
Reissman, Catherine Kohler. 1983. "Women and Medicalization: A New
  Perspective." *Social Policy* 14:3–18.
Romalis, Shelley, ed. 1982. *Childbirth: Alternatives to Medical Control.* Austin:
  University of Texas Press.
Rothman, Barbara Katz. 1982. *In Labor: Women and Power in the Birthplace.*
  New York: W. W. Norton.
——— 1986. *The Tentative Pregnancy: Prenatal Diagnosis and the Future of
  Motherhood.* New York: Viking Penguin.
——— 1989. *Recreating Motherhood: Ideology and Technology in Patriarchal Society.*
  New York: W. W. Norton.
———, ed. 1993. *The Encyclopedia of Childbearing.* New York: Henry Holt.
Rushing, Elizabeth. 1988. "Midwifery and the Sources of Occupational
  Autonomy." Ph.D. diss., Duke University.
——— 1993. "Ideology in the Reemergence of North American Midwifery."
  Work and Occupations 20 (1): 46–67.
Salazar, Claudia. 1991. "A Third World Woman's Text: Between the Politics of
  Criticism and Cultural Politics." In *Women's Words,* ed. Gluck and Patai,
  93–106.
Sargent, Carolyn. 1989. *Maternity, Medicine, and Power: Reproductive Decisions in
  Urban Benin.* Berkeley: University of California Press.
Sawicki, Jana. 1991. *Disciplining Foucault.* New York: Routledge.
Scheper-Hughes, Nancy, and Margaret Lock. 1991. "The Message in the
  Bottle: Illness and the Micropolitics of Resistance." *Journal of Psychohistory*
  18 (4): 409–32.
Scott, Joan. 1991. "The Evidence of Experience." *Critical Inquiry* 17:773–97.
Sharpe, Joanne. 1996. "Gendering Nationhood." In *BodySpace,* ed. Duncan,
  97–108.
Sharpe, Mary. 1998. "Ontario Midwifery in Transition: An Exploration of
  Midwives' Perceptions of the Impact of Midwifery Legislation in its First
  Year." In Shroff, ed., *The New Midwifery,* 201–44.
Shiva, Vandana. 1988. *Staying Alive: Women, Ecology, and Development.* London:
  Zed.
Shroff, Farah, ed. 1998. *The New Midwifery in Canada: Reflections on Renaissance
  and Regulation.* Toronto: Women's Press.

Shuttleworth, Joanne. 2002. "Hospital Manager Says Disputes Being Ironed Out." *Guelph Daily Mercury,* June 13.

Sleep, J., J. Roberts, and I. Chalmers. 1989. "The Second Stage of Labour." In *A Guide to Effective Care in Pregnancy and Childbirth,* ed. M. Enkin, M. Keirse, and I. Chalmers, 1129–44. Oxford: Oxford University Press.

Spain, Daphne. 1992. *Gendered Spaces.* Chapel Hill: University of North Carolina Press.

Spivak, Gayatri Chakravorty. 1993. *Outside in the Teaching Machine.* London: Routledge.

Stabile, Carol. 1994. *Feminism and the Technological Fix.* Manchester: Manchester University Press.

Stacey, Judith. 1991. "Can There Be a Feminist Ethnography?" In *Women's Words,* ed. Gluck and Patai, 111–20.

Stanley, Liz, and Sue Wise. 1990. *Feminist Praxis.* London: Routledge and Kegan Paul.

Stewart, Kathleen. 1990. "Backtalking the Wilderness: Appalachian Engenderings." In *Uncertain Terms,* ed. Ginsberg and Lowenhaupt-Tsing, 43–56.

Strathern, Marilyn. 1992. *After Nature: English Kinship in the Late 20th Century.* Cambridge: Cambridge University Press.

Sullivan, Deborah, and Rose Weitz. 1988. *Labor Pains: Modern Midwives and Home Birth.* New Haven: Yale University Press.

Susie, Debra. 1987. *In the Way of Our Grandmothers: A Cultural View of Twentieth Century Midwifery in Florida.* Athens: University of Georgia Press.

Sutton, Wendy. 1996. "The Saga of the Toronto Birth Centre." *Health Law Journal* 4:151–78.

Taylor, Janelle, Linda Lane, and Danielle Wosniack, eds. 2004. *Consuming Motherhood.* New Brunswick, NJ: Rutgers University Press.

Thacker, S. B., and D. F. Stroup. 1999. Continuous electronic fetal heart rate monitoring versus intermittent auscultation for assessment during labor. Cochrane Library. Issue 1. Oxford.

Thomas, Nicholas. 1996. "Cold Fusion." *American Anthropologist* 98 (1): 9–25.

Trevathan, Wenda. 1984. *Human Birth: An Evolutionary Perspective.* New York: Aldine de Gruyter.

Tuana, Nancy. 1989. "The Weaker Seed: The Sexist Bias of Reproductive Theory." In *Feminism and Science,* ed. Nancy Tuana. 147–71. Bloomington: Indiana University Press.

Tyson, Holliday. 1991. "Outcomes of 1,001 Midwife Attended Home Births in Toronto, 1983 to 1988." *Birth* 18 (1): 14–19.

Van Hollen, Cecilia. 2003. *Birth on the Threshold: Childbirth and Modernity in South India.* Berkeley: University of California Press.

Van Wagner, Vicki. 1988. "Women Organizing for Midwifery in Ontario." *Resources for Feminist Research* 17 (3): 115–18.

——— 1991. "With Women: Community Midwifery in Ontario." Master's thesis, York University.

——— 2004. "Why Legislation? Using Regulation to Strengthen Midwifery in Ontario." In *Reconceiving Midwifery,* ed. Bourgeault, Benoit, and Davis-Floyd, 71–90.

Visweswaran, Kamala. 1994. *Fictions of Feminist Ethnography.* Minneapolis: University of Minnesota Press.

Wedenoja, William. 1989. "Mothering and the Practice of Balm in Jamaica." In *Women as Healers,* ed. C. McClain, 76–97.

Wertz, Richard, and Dorothy Wertz. 1989. *Lying-In: A History of Childbirth in America.* New Haven: Yale University Press.

Wiegers, T., M. Keirse, J. van der Zee, and G. Berghs. 1996. "Outcome of Planned Home and Planned Hospital Births in Low Risk Pregnancies: Prospective Study in Midwifery Practices in the Netherlands." *BMJ* 313:1309–13.

Yanagisako, Sylvia, and Carole Delaney, eds. 1995. *Naturalizing Power.* London: Routledge.

Index